What People Are Saying about
Heart Smarter for Women

"We have been advocates for women's health for many years. Our goal is to ensure that all women understand that heart disease is different in women. Women should have access to the knowledge, the services, and the tools to live long, healthy lives. *Heart Smarter for Women* is an important resource for women of all ages who want to take the journey to living a more heart-healthy life. With real-life, practical advice on everything from nutrition information to sleep habits and stress management to finding a true physician partner, *Heart Smarter for Women* teaches women how to be proactive about their health and take the small steps that will have a huge impact on their heart health."

Iris and Saul Katz
Cofounders, Katz Institute for Women's Health, Northwell Health

"Self-management and patient/provider partnerships are pivotal for the heart health of women. Drs. Mieres and Rosen have provided women the impetus, resources, and skill sets for this momentous undertaking."

Nanette K. Wenger, MD, MACC, MACP, FAHA
Professor of Medicine (Cardiology) Emeritus,
Emory University School of Medicine
Founding Consultant, Emory Women's Heart Center

"As women work so hard to make their mark in a competitive world, one place we're overtaking men is in heart disease. This book is a must-have for every woman to make her heart health a priority while she soars in life."

Deborah Roberts
Senior National Affairs Correspondent, ABC News

Heart Smarter for Women should be required reading for all women who want to live a long and healthy life. The information presented provides women with the tools and encouragement to protect and preserve their heart health. Women who follow the simple steps outlined here will thrive! Grab a copy now for every woman you love."

Celina Gorre
CEO, WomenHeart

"This book is a must-read for every woman who wants to maximize her heart health, especially those for whom it is difficult to find a starting point. Demystifying complex information and providing simple tools and steps every woman can take to achieve better heart health are two challenges that *Heart Smarter for Women* successfully takes on. The six-step program outlined in this book will put you well on your way to understanding the why and the how of better heart health!"

Tara Narula, MD, FACC
Associate Professor of Cardiovascular Medicine, Zucker School of Medicine, Hofstra/Northwell
Senior Medical Correspondent, CBS News

"*Heart Smarter for Women* is the GPS for women to most efficiently optimize their heart health and that of their families and communities."

C. Noel Bairey Merz, MD, FACC, FAHA, FESC
Professor of Medicine and Director, Barbra Streisand Women's
Heart Center and Preventive Cardiac Center, Smidt Heart Institute
at Cedars-Sinai Medical Center

"Finally a book that not only offers information on *what* to do but *how* to do the things that can actually make a difference and save your life. In *Heart Smarter for Women*, Drs. Mieres and Rosen give women and their families the tools to take the simple steps to heart-healthy living. This book is a much-needed guide to heart health for all women in America today, and it will truly change your life."

Jane Hanson
Media and Presentation Coaching

"Heart disease is the number-one cause of death for women, and still too few women know this. Heart disease in women is under-researched, underdiagnosed, and undertreated. All women should read *Heart Smarter for Women*. It will empower them to understand and reduce their risk of heart disease. Everything you do that is good for your heart is good for the rest of you. Drs. Mieres and Rosen, world-class experts, share their knowledge in a straightforward and engaging way. Buy one for you, and buy one for a woman you love."

Holly S. Andersen, MD, FACC
The Ronald O. Perelman Heart Institute
The New York Presbyterian Hospital

"Prevention of cardiac events and controlling heart disease risk factors have been a personal struggle for many years. In partnership with the team at the Katz Institute for Women's Health, I followed the simple steps in *Heart Smarter for Women*, set manageable goals, and now, just a few months later, I have significantly decreased my risk for heart disease by having heart-healthy numbers. This book is a must-read for all women who wish to have a healthier heart."

Kathy Khodadadi
Women's Heart Health Program participant at the
Katz Institute for Women's Health

"*Heart Smarter for Women* offers the basis to change lives and improve human health by providing the essential tools to empower women to take the simple steps needed to prevent and control heart disease."

Roxana Mehran, MD, FACC, FACP, FCCP, FESC, FAHA, FSCAI
Professor of Medicine (Cardiology), Director of Interventional Cardiovascular Research and Clinical Trials, Icahn School of Medicine at Mount Sinai

"Several years ago, I experienced a rare form of heart attack. My successful recovery was due to two brilliant and dedicated women cardiologists—Drs. Stacey Rosen and Jennifer Mieres. They each partnered with me and played an important role, guiding and teaching me how to live a heart-healthy life, all of which is now captured in this wonderful book, *Heart Smarter for Women*. Their real and common-sense suggestions, their thoughtfulness, and their way of just simply encouraging and *loving* me brought me to my happy place. I now pay it forward, inspired and mentored by Drs. Rosen and Mieres, as a WomenHeart Champion, facilitating a support group for women living with or at risk of heart disease."

Joyce Lenard
WomenHeart Champion

"Heart Smarter for Women is a must-read for women as well as their healthcare professionals. The book provides a roadmap for simple lifestyle changes that, as physicians, we should all be recommending to the women in our care. It is an armamentarium for members of the healthcare community who want to ensure that their female patients are living the most heart-healthy life possible. An added benefit is that, because women are the drivers of overall family health, women following the six-week program will likely make their entire families healthier."

Lawrence Smith, MD, MACP
Founding Dean, Zucker School of Medicine, Hofstra/Northwell

"Heart Smarter for Women is a guide made for every woman. Drs. Mieres and Rosen have developed a six-week program that will help you understand if you are at risk for heart disease and empower you to take control of your own heart health. This book is the first step to improve the dialogue between women and their physicians, with the goal of identifying risk factors for heart disease, reducing heart disease, and ultimately saving more women's lives."

Martha Gulati, MD, MS, FACC, FAHA, FASPC, FESC
Author of *Saving Woman's Hearts*

"As a pediatric cardiologist, I know that heart disease in women has very early roots—from family risk factors to dietary habits and lifestyle choices. Drs. Mieres and Rosen provide clear guidance on the important steps that women of all ages can take to ensure a heart-healthy future. If an ounce of prevention is worth a pound of cure, then women who read this wonderful book will quickly realize that it is worth its weight in gold."

Angela Romano, MD
Pediatric Cardiologist, Cohen Children's Medical Center,
Northwell Health

"Drs. Mieres and Rosen are a dynamic duo of female cardiologists who genuinely want to help decrease heart disease in women. With the help of Lori Russo, JD, and Marissa Licata, RD, their new book is a must-read for all women to prevent or manage heart disease. People have different tastes in food, different budgets, and different situations; the book gives a variety of simple options to stay heart healthy. There are several books written on how to stay heart healthy, but this comprehensive book stands out since it is not just about exercising and what you eat; it is a holistic approach to living a healthy and happy life, free of the complications of heart disease. I will recommend this book to all of my patients!"

Annabelle Santos Volgman, MD, FACC, FAHA
McMullan-Eybel Endowed Chair in Clinical Cardiology
Professor of Medicine, Medical Director, Heart Center for Women,
Rush College of Medicine

"In this essential guide, Drs. Mieres and Rosen offer up easy tips and tools that help women adopt a heart-healthy lifestyle. Their philosophy? Even the smallest steps can make a big difference—and save a life. *Heart Smarter for Women* should be every woman's companion on the journey to heart health."

Susan Spencer
SVP, Subject Matter
Former Editor-in-Chief, *Woman's Day* magazine

"*Heart Smarter for Women* is a meticulously researched and beautifully written guide to achieving heart health. It champions a unique program that promotes lifelong healthy choices using techniques that every woman can embrace, regardless of age."

Penny Stern, MD, MPH, FACPM, FACOEM
Chief, Preventive & Lifestyle Medicine, Occupational Medicine,
Epidemiology & Prevention,
Katz Institute for Women's Health

"The most comprehensive lifestyle plan for optimal heart health tailored to the unique needs of women that I have read. *Heart Smarter for Women* offers a straightforward and easy-to-follow approach for creating a healthy lifestyle, reducing stress, improving your diet, and exercising effectively. Importantly, this book is written by leading authorities in the field of cardiovascular prevention and women's health. This book stands above all others as the book to have and to use as a guide to make important and positive heart-healthy changes in your life."

Leslee J. Shaw, PhD, FACC, FAHA, MSCCT
Chair and Professor of Women's Health
Director, Blavatnik Family Women's Health Research Institute,
Icahn School of Medicine at Mount Sinai

HEART

smarter

FOR WOMEN

HEART
smarter
FOR WOMEN

SIX WEEKS TO
a healthier heart

JENNIFER H. MIERES, MD, FACC

STACEY E. ROSEN, MD, FACC

WITH LORI M. RUSSO, JD

AND MARISSA LICATA, MS, RD

Advantage®

Published by Advantage, Charleston, South Carolina.
Member of Advantage Media Group.

ADVANTAGE is a registered trademark, and the Advantage colophon is a trademark of Advantage Media Group, Inc.

Printed in the United States of America.

10 9 8 7 6 5 4 3 2 1

ISBN: 978-1-64225-246-0
LCCN: 2021925603

Exercise photos provided by Onward Publishing, Inc.

This publication is designed to provide accurate and authoritative information in regard to the subject matter covered. It is sold with the understanding that the publisher is not engaged in rendering legal, accounting, or other professional services. If legal advice or other expert assistance is required, the services of a competent professional person should be sought.

 Advantage Media Group is proud to be a part of the Tree Neutral® program. Tree Neutral offsets the number of trees consumed in the production and printing of this book by taking proactive steps such as planting trees in direct proportion to the number of trees used to print books. To learn more about Tree Neutral, please visit **www.treeneutral.com**.

Advantage Media Group is a publisher of business, self-improvement, and professional development books and online learning. We help entrepreneurs, business leaders, and professionals share their Stories, Passion, and Knowledge to help others Learn & Grow. Do you have a manuscript or book idea that you would like us to consider for publishing? Please visit **advantagefamily.com**.

To all of the strong women in our lives who have partnered with us on this journey, from whom we continue to learn each and every day. We do this for you and for the next generation of women who will stand on your shoulders.

Contents

PART ONE: WOMEN AND HEART DISEASE—AN OVERVIEW

PART TWO: SIX S.T.E.P.S. IN SIX WEEKS TO A HEALTHIER HEART

PART THREE: GET SMARTER—ELEVATE YOUR HEART IQ

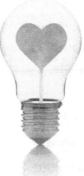

Acknowledgments

Completing *Heart Smarter for Women: Six Weeks to a Healthier Heart*, which is an updated edition of our previous book, *Heart Smart for Women*, was made possible through the continued support and encouragement of so many!

We want to take this opportunity to acknowledge and offer a heartfelt thanks to the village of women and men who inspired, assisted, and, most importantly, cheered us on to the finish line.

To our remarkable, resilient patients, you are the reason we continue to be passionate about empowering women of all ages and backgrounds to take an active role in optimizing their health and to be their own best advocates. Each of your stories, questions, and concerns has been what drives us to continue our journey toward providing you with a simple plan for heart-healthy living. You are at the forefront of all we do.

We want to acknowledge those who helped us make *Heart Smarter for Women* a reality. A sincere thanks to our cowriters Lori M. Russo, JD, and Marissa Licata, RD. Lori, again, worked tirelessly to bring this book to completion. Her guidance, insight as a skilled patient advocate, and expertise were invaluable. Marissa successfully updated our nutrition chapters with an eye toward advances in nutrition science related to heart health. She created a plan that is practical and easy to follow.

Heartfelt gratitude, again, to Dr. Jennifer Ashton for her thoughtful and insightful foreword and for being a powerful voice as a physician and health advocate in the effort to expand health education for women.

Thanks to Heather Wagner for her insights and timely and superb feedback on the manuscript, as well as to Nate Best, Kristin Goodale, Megan Elger, and the team at Advantage Media Group|ForbesBooks for their guidance, feedback, and expertise. Our colleagues at the Katz Institute for Women's Health provided invaluable support and encouragement. Catherine Blotiau, Emilie Blotiau, Kaye-Lani Brissett, Rosemarie Ennis, Lisa Fisher, Reva Gajer, Lori Ginsberg, Gail Greenwood, Dr. Bella Grossman, Elaine Ianazzi, Leslie Kang, Marlena Krispin, Rosagna Mancebo, Kim McHugh, Dr. Beth Nash, Dorraine Russin, Dr. Penny Stern, Alexa Tiven, and Sharon Zarabi: We are truly blessed to work alongside all of you each and every day. And to our friends at the Center for Wellness and Integrative Medicine: Lisa Bondy, Jennifer Caliendo, Tina Conroy, Deborah McElligott, Deborah DiMisa, and Ashley Tam.

A world of thanks to our team members in the Center for Equity of Care: Anu Anish, Neela Gomes, Richard LaRochelle, Cynthia Lewin, Lori Loose, Dr. Johanna Martinez, Dr. Elizabeth Maltin, Dr. Elizabeth McCulloch, Samantha Rosario, Colleen Ruggiero, and Tish Walsh.

Special thanks to Iris and Saul Katz for their visionary approach to women's health and their commitment to empowering women to focus on prevention and wellness. We are honored to join you in this effort. This book would not have been possible without your foresight and strong support.

Thank you to Nanci and Larry Roth and the Roth Family Foundation for their generosity and support of the Women's Heart Program at Northwell. Through the program we are able to provide personalized care for the prevention, early detection, and treatment of cardiovascular disease in women. Thank you to Dr. Jeffrey Kuvin, the chairman of Northwell's Department of Cardiology, for his encouragement and support of expanding our mission to improve the heart health of women through expanded clinical programs, education, research, and advocacy.

As longtime physicians at Northwell Health, we are indebted to our colleagues for embracing the need to see women's health differently. Thanks to our leadership team and colleagues: Michael Dowling, Mark Solazzo, Dr. Larry Smith, Dr. David Battinelli, Dr. Jill Kalman, Ralph Nappi, Terry Lynam, Kevin Beiner, Stephen Bello, Dr. Christina Brennan, Dr. Jean Cacciabaudo, Maxine Carrington, Donna Drummond, Victoria Faustini, Alice Fornari, Dr. Eugenia Gianos, Dr. Kathy Gallo, Rebecca Gordon, Dr. Evelina Grayver, Dr. Sonia Henry, Dr. Barry Kaplan, Dr. Stanley Katz, Jeffrey Kraut, Brian Lally, Robert Lane, Phyllis McCready, Joe Moscola, Dr. Jason Naidich, Dr. Ira Nash, Dr. Deb Salas-Lopez, Deborah Schiff, Joe Schulman, Dr. Varinder Singh, Susan Somerville, Ramon Soto, Eugene Tangney, Bessy Thangavelu, Chantal Weinhold, Maureen White, Dr. Abbey Wolf, Dr. Andrew Yacht, as well as the Katz Institute for Women's Health Clinical Steering Committee and the rest of our Northwell family.

Our friends at the American Heart Association have provided continued words of encouragement as well as the opportunity to meet many of the women who inspired us to write this book. Nancy Brown, Julie Del Barto, Sue Flor, Leslie Holland, Brooks Lancaster, Kathy

Munsch, Jaimie Racanelli, Nicole Sapio: You have been with us every step of the way. A special thank you to our friends at WomenHeart for overseeing a comprehensive program of uniquely patient-centered initiatives, including Celina Gore and the physician members of the Scientific Advisory Council. We are grateful for the work of the many WomenHeart champions who volunteer to educate, support, and advocate for women with or at risk for heart disease.

We are fortunate to have a continually expanding network of cardiology colleagues who are luminaries in their respective fields, collaborators, and innovators on the journey to gender equity and women's heart health. We want to thank the incomparable Dr. Nanette Wenger, our hero and mentor, and the champions of women's health, Drs. Niti Aggarwal, Holly Andersen, Noel Bairey Merz, Robert Bonow, Martha Gulati, Sharonne Hayes, Alice Jacobs, Michelle Johnson, Sandra Lewis, Gina Lundberg, Laxmi Mehta, Erin Michos, Virginia Miller, Blijian Parapid, Cheryl Pegus, Lawrence Phillips, Ileana Pina, Rita Redberg, Robert Roswell, Garima Sharma, Leslee Shaw, Toniya Singh, Allison Spatz, Annabelle Volgman, Mary (Minnow) Walsh, and Malissa Wood.

It is difficult to find the right words with which to thank our families. Our parents, sisters, brothers, husbands, and children have been there for us at every turn and have inspired and encouraged us to make the concept for this book a reality. To our remarkable, inspirational mothers, Jean Mieres, Harriet Rosen, Rae Russo, and Marie Tantillo; Aunt Barbara Mieres; and our siblings, Jackie Mieres Johnston, Arlene Mieres Franzcak, Anne Russo Meyer, Fred Rosen, and Stuart Russo: You have been our role models, our sounding boards, and our best cheerleaders.

Most of all, we wish to thank our husbands, Drs. Haskel Fleishaker, Mark Silverman, Barry Shpizner, and John Licata and our children, Zoë Mieres Fleishaker; Max, Rebecca, and Sarah Silverman; Julia Posluns; Mark and Jeremy Shpizner; Alisan Oliver-Li; Ella Radcliffe; and Gia and Lucas Licata. Without your encouragement, understanding, support, and love we would not have been successful in this major and important accomplishment.

Foreword

The past three years have brought us to a critical juncture in health-care, where a redesign, reset, and creation of a "new normal" are essential to improving our health. As we learn to adapt to the new normal brought on by the COVID pandemic, it is abundantly clear that the more resilient we are, the better prepared we are to meet any challenges that come our way. The more tools we have in our arsenal to make us more resilient, the more prepared we will be. *Heart Smarter for Women: Six Weeks to a Healthier Heart* is one such tool.

Health disparities and inequities unmasked by COVID-19 have taught us that the pandemic affects women's health in a multitude of ways. In addition to the threat to women's physical health, women have been negatively impacted on psychological, emotional, social, and financial levels as well. And the focus on COVID has caused many of us to put other health issues on hold or push concerns aside. This is especially troublesome and dangerous, as we know from recent studies that, despite decades of grassroots campaigns which have raised awareness about the magnitude of cardiovascular disease in women, there has not been a corresponding decrease in the numbers of women with cardiovascular disease.

Consider this: Although heart disease is the leading cause of death in women, statistics show that the number of women who know that it is their greatest personal health risk has actually significantly *decreased over the past decade! Awareness has gone from an all-time high of 65 percent to a current state of 44* percent! We have to act now!

Heart disease in women is underdiagnosed and underresearched, so it's significant to receive such conclusive medical insight from Drs. Mieres and Rosen, leading cardiologists with over fifty years of combined experience in cardiovascular medicine.

One of the reasons that some ignore personal health is because it demands a change that can at times be daunting. Another reason is that we simply don't understand how our bodies work nor where we should start with lifestyle changes. *Heart Smarter for Women* helps us navigate through an evidence-based blueprint for personal implementation and rules out any reluctance we might have on how to begin this journey. This book is a well-rounded resource that demystifies the science, biology, and statistics about our bodies and translates its meaning into clear, simple steps that make changing habits doable. The "heart smarter" program Drs. Mieres and Rosen provide is effective, practical, and sustainable.

As a woman, a physician, and the daughter of a cardiologist, I recognize the importance of heart disease prevention and awareness ... especially for women. There is an urgent need for better communication of critical information, and no one does this better than Drs. Mieres and Rosen et al. There are many good books on this topic, but this one truly could save your life.

As women, we need to learn how to be more resilient and how to translate that into action. There are solutions that can help us achieve the level of resiliency, self-care, and wellness we all deserve. The great thing is that this can be an exciting journey! Let this book be the turning point to making your health a priority. Find the courage to take the steps needed toward heart-healthy living and do it the "heart smarter" way!

Jennifer Ashton, MD, MS, FACOG, OB-GYN
ABC News Chief Women's Health Correspondent

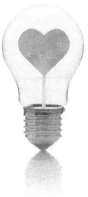

Important Note to the Reader

This book is for informational purposes only and is not intended to take the place of medical advice from a trained medical professional. You are advised to consult a doctor or qualified health professional before acting on any of the information in this book.

Introduction

This is a book for every woman.

No matter who you are, you can make it your mission to become smarter about your heart health.

This book is written for you, designed to empower you with the knowledge and tools you'll need to lead a healthier life.

Heart disease is the number one killer of women. Yet far too few women recognize its risks, and there have been tremendous disparities in how women are diagnosed and treated.

Some of our earlier writings focused on the abysmally low awareness about heart health in Black and Latina women, as revealed in a publication by the American Heart Association. Our goal was to show that heart disease is preventable.

In response to statistics from the American Heart Association showing an increase in the number of women under the age of fifty-five dying from heart disease, many of whom didn't recognize that heart disease was their number one risk for death and disability, we broadened our message to share important research with all women about how to live heart-healthier lives.

We have received enthusiastic feedback from readers who have welcomed this knowledge and have made significant changes in their lives—changes that have dramatically improved their health.

But we want to do more. We want to reach every woman with the powerful message that making a few simple changes will have lasting impact on their heart health. So we wrote a book that all women can use as a call to action and as a guide to demystify the facts about heart disease.

That knowledge is especially critical for a new generation of women—women just like you. A ten-year study from the American Heart Association shows that women's awareness of the risks of heart disease has declined dramatically in the past decade, with fewer than half of all women recognizing that heart disease is their leading killer. The greatest declines in awareness were among women under the age of thirty-five as well as among Black and Latina women.[1]

The latest research demonstrates precisely how critical it is for you to become heart smarter. A May 2021 study from the *Lancet* discovered that despite decades of campaigns designed to raise awareness of the impact of cardiovascular disease in women, it remains understudied, underrecognized, underdiagnosed, and undertreated.[2] The Lancet Commission has announced ambitious goals to reduce the

---

1   American Heart Association, "Heart Disease Awareness Decline Spotlights Urgency to Reach Younger Women and Women of Color," September 21, 2020, https://newsroom.heart.org/news/heart-disease-awareness-decline-spotlights-urgency-to-reach-younger-women-and-women-of-color.

2   Birgit Vogel, MD, et al., "The Lancet Women and Cardiovascular Disease Commission: Reducing the Global Burden by 2030," *Lancet*, May 16, 2021, https://www.thelancet.com/journals/lancet/article/PIIS0140-6736%2821%2900684-X/fulltext.

burden of cardiovascular disease by 2030, with specific recommendations to ensure that women are better educated on ways to prevent heart disease. It is particularly critical to reach groups that are not traditionally regarded as being at high risk, such as young women—a group in which smoking rates and heart attacks are increasing.

This book is your invitation to become *heart smarter*—to combat statistics with knowledge and understanding. We want to partner with you as you begin the journey to heart health, providing you with clear, simple instructions and a six-week plan that has proven highly successful with readers and with our patients. We want to share new research and new guidelines that have been released since the publication of our previous book, *Heart Smart for Women*—information that will clarify how and why heart health matters for you. And we want to celebrate with you as you become a better partner to your doctor, as you stock your pantry with healthier items and prepare delicious healthy meals, as you try out new approaches to heart-healthy living.

These are choices that will impact not only your heart but your overall health. The steps we recommend in this book may also contribute to better gastrointestinal health, to lowered rates of dementia and improved cognitive abilities—to healthier aging. These are steps that can lengthen your life span and improve your energy.

This is your book, your guide to taking charge of your health in easy but meaningful ways.

You can do this. Start with one step, then another. Small steps that will make a big difference. Small steps that will make you smarter about your heart and your health.

Your Guide to Good Health

We have all heard the adage "If you have your health, you have everything." This bit of timeless wisdom often gets lost in or pushed aside by demands of our busy lives. But good health should be a priority. It is something we must consciously work for by taking control of our lives and putting ourselves first. Yet women often put themselves last, considering the needs of their family and friends above their own.

We want to help you break this cycle. We want to encourage you to recognize that your health matters. Our goal is to equip you with the tools you'll need and the knowledge that will place you firmly on the road to living a heart-healthy life.

Drs. Mieres and Rosen each have more than thirty years of medical experience in the field of cardiology, and we all share a passion for educating and empowering women to be active participants and effective advocates for their health.

This book is a call to action for women everywhere. More than 90 percent of all women have one or more risk factors of heart disease, but these risk factors can be acknowledged and addressed. We want to empower you with positive inspiration, because heart disease is largely preventable! In fact, research has shown that women can lower their risk of heart disease by as much as 80 percent simply by making healthy lifestyle changes. This can be anything from choosing to move every day to increasing your sleep to decreasing the amount of unhealthy fats in your daily diet. Any type of daily exercise, combined with small but mean-

OUR GOAL IS TO EQUIP YOU WITH THE TOOLS YOU'LL NEED AND THE KNOWLEDGE THAT WILL PLACE YOU FIRMLY ON THE ROAD TO LIVING A HEART-HEALTHY LIFE.

ingful changes in your daily food choices and your lifestyle, can have a tremendous impact on your health.

Awareness. Simple lifestyle changes. Forming a true partnership with your doctor. These are the key elements of heart health. Yet these elements so often elude us. We think we are too busy, too set in our ways, too old, or too young to form new habits and learn new approaches to preventing, minimizing, or reversing heart disease. But recent advances in the medical and scientific communities demonstrate that the opposite is true. It is never too soon or too late to adopt heart-healthy habits.

Our program will enable you to simply and easily begin to live a healthier life. If you follow our Six S.T.E.P.S. in Six Weeks to a Healthier Heart, by the end of those six weeks, the new behaviors you have learned will have become habits. And these habits will put you well on your way to living a heart-healthy life.

Heart disease is an equal opportunity killer, and so this book is for all women, from all walks of life, of all ages and all ethnicities. Heart disease continues to be the leading cause of death of women in the United States. It claims significantly more lives than all cancers combined. But the amazing fact is that over 80 percent of all heart disease is preventable! Great strides have been made in the prevention, early diagnosis, and treatment of heart disease in women. Yet awareness of these facts is not enough. Knowledge must be translated into action, and without simple lifestyle changes and strong doctor-patient partnerships, these strides will not translate into actual lives saved.

We have met women with heart disease or risk factors for heart disease who are eager to make heart-smart changes in their lives but don't know how to begin. The answer is right here, right now. Our mission is to demystify the science, the biology, and the statistics surrounding heart disease and to provide concrete, simple steps to begin the journey.

Heart Smarter for Women will help you understand the science behind heart disease, provide simple lifestyle changes you can make in your approach to eating, cooking, and exercising, and also offer concrete suggestions on how to develop the most effective partnership with your doctor. All of these things will help you address your risk factors for heart disease and improve the quality of your daily living.

We want you to continue to enjoy the foods you love, but we have highlighted simple changes to recipes, ingredients, and portion sizes that will yield a healthier version of those foods. You will find ways to maintain control of what you eat when eating out as well as when dining at home. You will also learn ways to incorporate exercise into your daily routine, even if you are convinced that you don't have an extra minute in your already jam-packed day.

We know our program works because we have seen the proof with our patients. We guarantee that with our six-week program you'll be on your way to living a heart-healthy life—moving more, eating better, living with less stress, and savoring life more.

About the Book

The more you know about the risks of heart disease and the simple but critical steps you can take to reduce your personal risk of developing heart disease, the more successful you will be on your journey to heart health. Toward that end, this book is separated into three parts.

Part one provides a comprehensive discussion of the workings of the healthy heart and the risk factors, signs, and symptoms of heart disease. We hope you find it enlightening! You may want to refer back to this section as needed. The important thing is that you familiarize yourself with the vocabulary of heart disease so that you can comfortably communicate with your doctor and advocate for your own healthcare. These chapters will help you identify and assess your own risk factors for developing heart disease so that you understand the special issues you may face. They will also provide the necessary background regarding the "whys" of our six-week program and explain how each step may apply to your particular health situation.

Part two provides the "how," with the complete Six S.T.E.P.S. in Six Weeks to a Healthier Heart Program. Here you will find a week-by-week road map for your journey to heart health, including choosing the right foods, dining at home and outside of the home, finding a doctor who is the right physician partner for you, and learning to maximize sleep and minimize stress.

Part three is new to this edition and contains helpful content designed to equip you to elevate your heart IQ and become smarter about your heart health. Here, you will find six access points you can use to immediately begin to incorporate your new knowledge into your daily life. There are opportunities to learn more with detailed portion size guidelines; training tips for strength and flexibility exercises you can practice in the comfort of your home; recovery tips for heart attack survivors; and answers to questions you may have about heart disease and heart treatments, tests, and medications, plus a week of easy and delicious menus to jump-start your goals for heart-healthy eating.

This book was inspired by the thousands of incredible women we have met as patients and at community lectures and health screenings over the past thirty years. It is meant to empower you and to translate the knowledge of heart disease into an action plan that will put you firmly on the road to a healthier heart.

JENNIFER H. MIERES, MD, FACC, FAHA
STACEY E. ROSEN, MD, FACC, FAHA
LORI M. RUSSO, JD

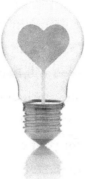

Overview

The more you know about heart disease and the simple but critical steps you can take to reduce your personal risk of developing heart disease, the more successful you will be on your journey to heart health. Toward that end, this book is separated into three parts:

Part One provides a comprehensive discussion of the workings of the healthy heart, risk factors, and signs and symptoms of heart disease. This information will give you the background information necessary to develop a familiarity with the workings of your heart! You may want to refer back to Part One as needed. The important thing is that you familiarize yourself with the vocabulary of heart disease so that you can comfortably communicate with your doctor and better advocate for your own healthcare.

Part One will help you identify and assess your own risk factors for developing heart disease so that you understand the special issues you may face. You will learn about risk factors that are unique or more important for women. It will also provide the necessary background regarding the "whys" of the Six Weeks to a Healthier Heart and how they may apply to your particular health situation.

Part Two provides the "how," with the complete Six S.T.E.P.S. in Six Weeks program. Here you will find a week-by-week roadmap for your journey to heart health, including choosing the right foods and dining at home and out of the home. With an emphasis on the importance of food choices for your heart health, you will also find practical nutritional information. You will learn about the power of partnerships, as well as possible approaches to finding a doctor who is the right physician-partner. Finally, we provide tips to help you learn to maximize sleep and manage stress.

Part Three provides a practical guide to meal planning to get you started, physical activity suggestions, a discussion of heart medications, treatments and tests, as well as advice for heart attack survivors, a Q&A section, and a helpful glossary.

PART ONE

WOMEN AND HEART DISEASE—AN OVERVIEW

*"When women take care of their health, they
become their own best friend."*
—MAYA ANGELOU

Chapter One

UNDERSTANDING HEART DISEASE IN WOMEN

As you begin your journey to a heart-healthier life, it's important to fully understand heart disease. Why does heart disease pose a specific risk for women—and why aren't more women talking about it?

We know that heart disease is an equal opportunity killer, and that over the past several decades it has been the number one cause of death of women in the United States—although fewer than half of American women identify it as such. The medical and scientific communities have gained tremendous insights into some of the unique health risks of women, and significant progress has been made toward reducing the number of women with heart disease. Yet every day there are women of varying backgrounds and ages whose stories tell us that there is much work to be done, women who remind us that we must all be vigilant about our own health and that the way to address our own risks of developing heart disease is to make simple lifestyle changes and establish a true partnership with our doctors, nurses, and healthcare team.

We want to introduce you to some of the women in our community. Their stories are different, their backgrounds diverse, yet they all have one important similarity.

Claudia is a forty-eight-year-old woman of Puerto Rican descent whose high-pressure job at a bank and busy family life keep her in a constant state of anxiety. She is often tired, experiences occasional heart palpitations, and sometimes feels as if she can't breathe.

Chandra is a thirty-three-year-old woman of South Asian descent who works as an assistant to the president of a small department store. Chandra has a history of elevated blood sugar and was recently diagnosed with type 2 diabetes.

Sasha is a fifty-nine-year-old Black woman who is trained as a physical therapist but now spends her days caring for her elderly mother at home. Recently, she has had several bouts of severe indigestion and nausea and an overwhelming cold and clammy feeling. She is coming down with flu.

Rebecca is a forty-two-year-old White woman who is a nurse on a cardiac unit of a large hospital. She has been extremely fatigued lately, although her schedule has not changed.

These four women have different life experiences, they represent different age brackets and ethnicities, and yet they are the same in one important respect. They all have signs and risk factors of heart disease.

We will follow these women more closely as we learn about their challenges and triumphs on their journeys to heart-smart living.

Let's begin with the story of Claudia, who works as a vice president at one of the country's leading banks. Claudia has a busy and full life. Since her promotion to VP five years ago, her daily work routine has been stressful, requiring long hours and frequent travel. In addition, her home life is quite active, as she and her husband have two teenage daughters with busy school and sports schedules of their own.

Claudia is very disciplined. She understands the importance of exercise and is careful to adhere to a daily exercise routine of a thirty-minute aerobic workout five days a week, combined with two days of strength training with light weights. But over the past two months, Claudia has noticed a change in her energy level. She is fatigued after only fifteen minutes on the treadmill. On weekends, while running her usual errands, she is dragging. She has begun making small changes to her routine to compensate, such as parking her car right next to the store entrance to minimize the walking distance to the store.

At first, Claudia assumed that her fatigue was a normal by-product of perimenopause; however, as the months have gone by, her low energy and fatigue have continued. She has noticed something else—something that is definitely out of character for her. Last month, during a particularly stressful period at work, she lost her temper with a colleague who was only doing his job in delivering some upsetting financial news. This colleague was only the messenger! Claudia was confused by her own behavior, as she has always prided herself on her ability to remain calm under pressure. In addition, she has experienced episodes of palpitations and a feeling of anxiety leading to left-upper-back pain.

Luckily for Claudia, it is time for her annual checkup where she has the chance to describe her symptoms to her doctor. Her doctor is concerned that Claudia's symptoms are consistent with heart disease.

What Is Heart Disease?

Heart disease, which is also sometimes referred to as cardiovascular disease, is an umbrella term that includes a range of diseases of the heart and blood vessels, including coronary artery disease, heart failure, heart valve conditions, and heart rhythm disturbances. This book will focus on a primary culprit of heart disease, atherosclerosis, the process whereby plaque, made up of substances that circulate in your blood, including calcium, fat, and cholesterol, builds up in the blood vessels, leading to the thickening and narrowing of the vessel walls. The buildup of plaque in the blood vessels that supply the heart can lead to a heart attack. Although heart disease is the focus of this book, our program is designed to prevent and control the risks for all conditions caused by atherosclerosis, which include heart attack and stroke. We mention heart attack and stroke together because your risk factors for heart disease also increase your chances of having a stroke. As you follow the program, you will not only be improving your heart and the vessels that supply it but also be positively affecting the blood vessels that supply your brain.

The Unique Challenge of Heart Disease

The fact that women are far more likely to die of heart disease than from all forms of cancer—in fact, heart disease remains the most common cause of death in women and men—is a clear indication of how important it is to know how to prevent or stop it. This can sometimes be difficult because heart disease can masquerade as indigestion, breathlessness, or general fatigue, thereby delaying early diagnosis. For women, heart disease can present with symptoms other than chest pain or chest pressure. It's important to remember these three facts:

- Heart disease can be difficult to diagnose in its early stages.

- Heart disease can develop silently over time; it does not always announce its presence and get you to seek treatment.

- Heart disease can build up over years, or sometimes decades, until it makes itself known (for many women that means beginning in their twenties!), often in the form of a heart attack or stroke.

But it does not have to be that way. Heart disease is largely preventable and treatable—and, as we go through the steps to heart health together, you will learn how to keep this most important organ healthy.

FOR WOMEN, HEART DISEASE CAN PRESENT WITH SYMPTOMS OTHER THAN CHEST PAIN OR CHEST PRESSURE.

Know the Facts

To get a clear understanding of where heart disease ranks in terms of women's health, here's a quick look at the numbers.

According to the American Heart Association[3]:

- **Nine out of ten** women have one or more risk factors for heart disease.

- **Nearly half** of all Black women aged twenty and older (49 percent) have heart disease.

- Hispanic women are likely to develop heart disease **ten years earlier** than non-Hispanics.

- **One in three** women will die of heart disease.

But:

- **One in eight** women will develop breast cancer.

---

3   "The Facts about Women and Heart Disease," Go Red for Women, accessed November 16, 2020, https://www.goredforwomen.org/en/about-heart-disease-in-women/facts.

- **One in twenty-six** women will die of breast cancer.

The Causes of Heart Disease: Men versus Women

Despite the perception of heart disease as a "man's disease," *women and men are at equal risk of developing heart disease and suffering a heart attack.* In fact, until 2013, more women died each year from heart disease than men—when the rates became equivalent![4] In addition, women face a 20 percent increased risk of developing heart failure or dying within five years after their first severe heart attack compared to men.

Despite the fact that women are at equal risk of heart attack and heart disease, until recently, most research and treatments have been focused on men. The medical and scientific communities have historically underestimated the prevalence and importance of heart disease in women. For many years, this resulted in a failure to study the differences in the way men and women develop and experience heart disease. In fact, it is only within the past two decades that the medical and scientific communities expanded their research focus to include all aspects of women's heart health, from risk factors to diagnosis to treatment.

There are certain risk factors that men and women share. These include smoking, high blood pressure (hypertension), diabetes, sedentary lifestyle, high cholesterol, and family history of heart problems. The more risk factors you have, regardless of whether you are a man or a woman, the greater your chances of having a heart

---

4   Justin A. Ezekowitz et al., "Is there a Sex Gap in Surviving an Acute Coronary Syndrome or Subsequent Development of Heart Failure?" *Circulation* December 8, 2020, https://www.ahajournals.org/doi/pdf/10.1161/CIRCULATIONAHA.120.048015.

attack or stroke. But there are important differences that are unique to and can be more dangerous for women:

- Women typically develop heart problems about seven to ten years later in life than men, but by about the age of sixty-five men and women suffer from heart disease at the same rate.

- Diabetes is a much more potent risk factor for women than for men. Diabetic women are three to seven times more likely to die from heart disease than diabetic men.

- Women tend to be more obese, more inclined to have a sedentary lifestyle, and more likely to suffer from hypertension and diabetes than men.

Certain conditions are considered to be "gender-specific" risk factors for heart disease and heart attacks in women. These include lupus or rheumatoid arthritis and other inflammatory or autoimmune disorders; radiation-induced heart disease and other cardiac issues related to breast cancer treatment; and behavioral health issues like stress, depression, and anxiety.

Women with pregnancy-related complications of gestational diabetes, hypertension, preeclampsia, eclampsia, and preterm delivery are at increased risk for heart disease five to fifteen years after delivery.

Women with early-onset menopause (i.e., before age forty) are at greater risk than other women due to an early loss of estrogen, which is cardioprotective.

The Added Risk for Women of Black, Latina, or South Asian Heritage

In addition to the risk factors for women mentioned earlier, Black women, Latina women, and women of South Asian descent have an even higher risk of heart disease than White women—as much as a 69 percent higher risk—due to their higher incidence of high blood pressure, obesity, physical inactivity, diabetes, and metabolic syndrome (a group of risk factors that includes increased amounts of abdominal fat, high blood pressure, high cholesterol levels, and insulin resistance or glucose intolerance). Studies show that these risk factors can be more potent and prevalent in these ethnic groups.

What Does This Mean for *Your* Heart Health?

Now you know the statistics and can see how many women just like you are affected by heart disease. But we want to stress a point we made earlier: more than 80 percent of a woman's chance of developing heart disease is preventable with early identification, modification of risk factors, and healthy life choices. Our goal is to give you the added knowledge you need to clearly understand the science behind heart disease and then enable you to make simple lifestyle changes to prevent or stop the development of this disease. You can continue to enjoy your traditional foods, but now you will have information on how to prepare meals in healthier ways. Some of you may wish to lose a few pounds, but even for those of you who don't, learning to control portion size is key not only to controlling your weight but also to keeping blood sugar and cholesterol levels within range. Moreover, you will learn that it is possible to reach and maintain a healthy weight without depriving yourself or going on a severely restrictive diet. We will also suggest how you can make simple changes to your daily routine to become more active. You'll be delighted and surprised at how these easy changes add up and ultimately lead to the major improvements necessary to keep yourself healthy.

This is not a solo effort. One goal of the Six S.T.E.P.S in Six Weeks Program is for you to share what you learn with your family and friends, thereby improving their health and ultimately helping to break the cycle of heart disease. *Prevention* is key. In addition, simple lifestyle changes make a huge impact in reducing risk.

For some of us, heart disease starts as early as our twenties and continues silently, slowly blocking the arteries with plaque buildup. Heart disease, as we now know, is different not only between women and men but also among women of different races.

In the chapters ahead, we'll share information that will be helpful as you assess your personal risks and identify steps you can take to improve your heart health. The data can be sobering, but knowledge is power. With a few simple steps, you have the ability to take control of your health and begin to understand how choices you make about exercise, diet, and even sleep can lead to a healthier you.

So, turn the page and get started as you discover how getting and staying healthy can be so much easier and more fun than you had ever imagined. Experience firsthand how following our program over the next six weeks can put you on a lifelong road to good health. We promise that you will feel better, look better, and have more energy while reversing the path of heart disease.

Jennifer and Stacey are cardiologists with over sixty years of combined experience in cardiovascular medicine, treating women of all races, ethnicities, and ages. Lori is a patient and health advocate with a firm commitment to advancing heart health and knowledge. Marissa is a registered dietitian with twenty-two years of experience helping people achieve nutritional wellness. Our program works, and we have thousands of success stories to prove it. But before you begin the Six S.T.E.P.S. in Six Weeks Program, it is important that you understand more about your heart and how it works.

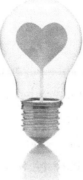

Chapter Two

THE HEALTHY HEART VERSUS THE DISEASED HEART

In chapter 1 we met Claudia, whose doctor expressed concern that the symptoms she was experiencing were consistent with heart disease. Claudia is surprised by this diagnosis—she prioritizes exercise and eating well and has not experienced chest pain or any of the symptoms that she thinks are signs of heart disease.

Like many women, Claudia is unaware of her risk factors for developing heart disease. She has regular mammograms and gets a flu shot every year, but this conversation with her doctor has prompted her to recognize that she needs to learn more—much more—about her heart.

In this chapter, we'll share this kind of knowledge. We'll explain how your heart works, what happens when it doesn't, and what the conditions are that lead to heart disease. This knowledge will help you put to use what you'll learn later in the book about keeping your heart healthy.

Although some of the information presented is fairly technical, please bear with us. It's important that you be familiar with the structure and workings of your heart along with the causes of problems. Use this chapter as a resource and refer back to it from time to time, because what might not make perfect sense now *will* later on as you build your heart knowledge and vocabulary. Now, let's learn anatomy!

Heart Anatomy

This first lesson in anatomy illustrates not only how the heart is constructed but how and why a healthy heart functions the way it does. Once you understand what the physical heart looks like inside and out, you will be able to envision how this hardworking organ goes about its job pumping life-giving blood through the body. You will also be able to visualize what actually happens to this amazing muscle when things go wrong.

The healthy heart is a simple and efficient fist-sized pump that sits in the center of your chest and beats approximately seventy-two times per minute, which is roughly one hundred thousand times every day. The heart's primary job is to pump nutrient-rich blood to all of the body's vital organs through a large set of tubes called arteries. Over the course of an average lifetime (approximately eighty-one years for White women, seventy-eight years for Black women, and eighty-four years for Hispanic women), the heart will beat more than three billion times without ever resting. Here's how it does it.

> OVER THE COURSE OF AN AVERAGE LIFETIME, THE HEART WILL BEAT MORE THAN THREE BILLION TIMES WITHOUT EVER RESTING.

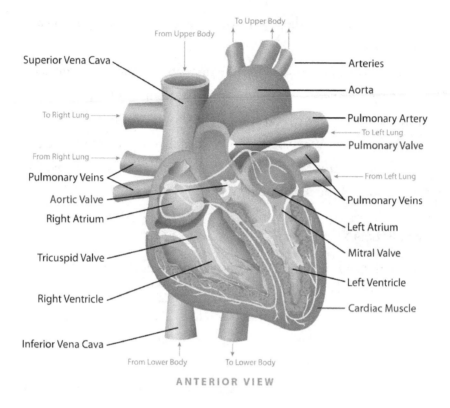

From Upper Body

To Upper Body

Superior Vena Cava

Arteries

Aorta

To Right Lung

Pulmonary Artery

To Left Lung

Pulmonary Valve

From Right Lung

From Left Lung

Pulmonary Veins

Pulmonary Veins

Aortic Valve

Right Atrium

Left Atrium

Tricuspid Valve

Mitral Valve

Right Ventricle

Left Ventricle

Cardiac Muscle

Inferior Vena Cava

From Lower Body

To Lower Body

ANTERIOR VIEW

TWO SIDES / FOUR CHAMBERS / FOUR VALVES

The heart is divided into two sides, separated by a wall called the *septum*. Each side has an upper and lower chamber, which are separated by structures called *valves*. The valves work like one-way doors that open to allow blood to flow through to the next chamber but close so the blood cannot flow backward. (It's the valves opening and closing that make the "lub-dub" sound, but more about this later.)

The right side of the heart pumps blood to the lungs, where it gets oxygen.

The left side of the heart receives the oxygen-rich blood from the lungs and pumps it throughout the body.

The atria are the upper two chambers. They collect blood flowing *into* the heart.

The ventricles are the lower two chambers. They pump blood *out* of the heart.

The tricuspid valve separates the right atrium and right ventricle.

The pulmonary valve separates the right ventricle and the pulmonary artery, which carries the blood to the lungs.

The mitral valve separates the left atrium and the left ventricle.

The aortic valve separates the left ventricle and the aorta, which pumps blood through the body.

ARTERIES AND VEINS

The arteries and veins are the major blood vessels that bring blood to and from the heart and deliver blood throughout the body.

The pulmonary artery carries blood to the lungs to pick up oxygen.

The aorta is the body's main artery and carries oxygen-rich blood to the body.

The pulmonary veins bring oxygen-rich blood from the lungs to the heart.

The superior and inferior vena cava are large veins that return the blood from the body back to the heart.

The coronary arteries get oxygen-rich blood from the aorta to the heart itself, which needs its own supply of blood to function.

HOW THE HEART WORKS

To give you a better idea of exactly how this miraculous pump works, let's follow the blood on its journey through the circulatory system.

Starting on the right side …

In search of oxygen, blood from the body comes into the heart through the *superior and inferior vena cava*, where it fills the *right atrium*.

The right atrium then contracts to open the *tricuspid valve* to allow this blood to move down into the *right ventricle.*

When the right ventricle is full, the tricuspid valve closes and the ventricle contracts to open the *pulmonary valve* so the blood can travel through the right and left *pulmonary arteries* to each lung for oxygen.

Returning on the left side …

This oxygenated blood then returns to the heart through the right and left *pulmonary veins,* where it fills the *left atrium.* The left atrium contracts to open the *mitral valve* and allow the blood to move into the *left ventricle.*

When the left ventricle is full, the mitral valve closes and the ventricle contracts to open the *aortic valve* so the oxygen-rich blood can travel into the *aorta* and throughout the body.

As is the case with all organs, the heart muscle also must receive oxygen-rich blood. This happens through the coronary arteries, which arise just past the aortic valve and run down the heart muscle, providing oxygen to the heart muscle itself.

THE SOUND OF YOUR HEARTBEAT

As we mentioned, the "lub-dub" sound that your doctor hears through the stethoscope is made when the heart valves open and close. It happens like this:

The "lub" sound comes from the closing of the mitral and tricuspid valves when the ventricles contract to pump blood out of the heart. The "dub" sound comes from the closing of the aortic and pulmonary valves when the ventricles relax to fill with blood from the atria.

Cardiac murmurs are extra sounds in between the "lub" and the "dub" that are heard with a stethoscope. Some murmurs may be related to normal flow of blood and are often called innocent or benign murmurs. But others may represent a range of heart abnormalities. If your healthcare professional detects a cardiac murmur, he or she will let you know if additional evaluation is recommended.

YOUR HEART'S ELECTRICAL SYSTEM

Along with the heart chambers, valves, and blood vessels, the heart has a sophisticated electrical system that produces the "spark" to drive the pumping of the heart. The heart contains an internal pacemaker and electrical circuits that allow it to work consistently and automatically over a lifetime.

This brief anatomy lesson offers a glimpse of how this amazing organ works and why it is so critical that you take care of it properly. Each component supports the heart's ability to function effectively; if any of the mechanical components becomes damaged or the blood vessels get clogged, the heart cannot work as it should.

Now let's take a closer look at what happens when the heart isn't functioning properly.

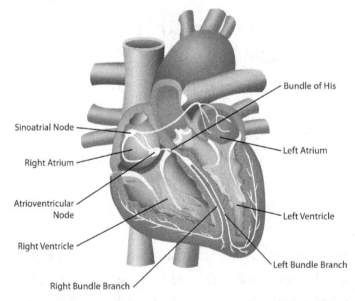

The normal heartbeat begins when the sinoatrial node produces an electrical signal. The electrical signal travels first through the two atria and then through the two ventricles via specialized wiring in the atria and the ventricles.

The Diseased Heart

Cardiovascular disease is a general term used to describe a range of diseases that affect the heart and blood vessels. These diseases can be related to the heart itself (a heart attack, heart failure, an electrical disorder); to the brain (a stroke); or to the blood vessels or circulatory systems that supply other critical organs (like the kidneys or extremities).

HEART ATTACK

Heart attack is the most common type of heart problem and occurs when the coronary arteries (the blood vessels that wrap around the surface of the heart and supply it with blood) are blocked enough to deprive the heart muscle of the blood it needs to function. If blood supply is limited for too long, the heart muscle will not recover, and this leads to the formation of a scar in part of the left ventricle. This is commonly related to coronary artery disease, which is due to blockages in the coronary arteries that can limit blood flow.

ISCHEMIC HEART DISEASE AND CORONARY ARTERY DISEASE

Ischemia (pronounced "is-key-me-uh") is the medical term describing an insufficient blood supply to nourish the organs of the body.

Coronary artery disease (CAD) is a form of ischemic heart disease where buildup of plaque and other blood-borne products leads to a narrowing of the lumen through which the blood flows. The heart muscle needs oxygen in order to function, and the coronary arteries are the pipes through which the blood transports that oxygen to the heart, like the pipes that transport water in your home. It's important that they remain open. This condition of plaque buildup is called *atherosclerosis*, commonly known as "hardening of the arteries." CAD can involve blockages that narrow the inside of blood vessels, but in its worst form, it can lead to a complete blockage where no blood flow can occur. A heart attack occurs when blood flow is severely limited or completely blocked.

In ischemic heart disease (IHD), inadequate blood supply to the heart muscle usually leads to symptoms such as shortness of breath; lightheadedness; chest pain or pressure (called angina); pain in the left arm or left shoulder, back, jaw, or throat; and heartburn or feelings of general fatigue. These symptoms can worsen during any type of exertion (exercise, climbing stairs, housework, etc.) or during times of emotional stress. Sometimes, however, this lack of adequate blood supply does not give rise to symptoms; that is, it can be "silent." Silent ischemia is said to occur when evidence of heart damage is found in the absence of the symptoms described above.

Although it was previously believed that atherosclerosis was the only process that caused ischemia, research to better understand IHD in women led to the appreciation that heart attacks can occur in the absence of atherosclerosis. Other abnormalities of blood vessels can also lead to heart attack, even in the absence of blockages. These include vessel spasm, microvascular dysfunction, spontaneous coronary artery dissection, and plaque rupture. These abnormalities can lead to the same types of symptoms and can cause heart muscle damage but without any blockages in the arteries.

ARRHYTHMIA

Arrhythmia describes an abnormal heart rhythm, or a heartbeat that is too slow, too fast, or irregular. Any irregular heartbeat will affect how efficiently the heart is working and how well blood is being pumped throughout the body.

If an arrhythmia is brief, it may be experienced as a skipped heartbeat and is generally nothing to be concerned about. However, a more worrisome form of arrhythmia can result in significant and long-lasting palpitations, lightheadedness, fainting, or even death.

HEART FAILURE

Heart failure is a misleading term, because the heart doesn't actually fail. Instead, it's more accurate to describe this as damage that results in the heart being unable to effectively pump blood to the entire body. The inability to pump efficiently leads to fluid buildup in the lungs and other tissues, with symptoms that include fatigue, shortness of breath, loss of appetite, nausea, and swollen feet and ankles. Heart failure is more common in women over the age of sixty and is often related to an underlying problem such as heart attack, high blood pressure, long-standing diabetes, or heart valve problems. Each year, more than one million women in the United States will develop heart failure. There is also a form of heart failure that younger women may develop during or shortly after pregnancy, called *peripartum cardiomyopathy*.

We now know that there is a form of heart failure where the heart pumps effectively but is less able to relax to allow blood to flow into the ventricles. This is called *heart failure with preserved ejection fraction (HFpEF)*. HFpEF is a more common form of heart failure in women than in men and has been found to be challenging to diagnose and treat. Approximately 61 to 76 percent of patients with HFpEF are women. Current research is focused on better ways to diagnose and treat this form of heart failure. Nonischemic heart failure (heart failure not related to ischemic heart disease) is more common in women than in men. This makes sense because diabetes, hypertension, and obesity are more prevalent in women, are stronger risk factors in women than in men, and, left undiagnosed or untreated, can ultimately lead to heart failure.

VALVULAR HEART DISEASE

Valvular heart disease occurs when there is an abnormality of any of the four heart valves that separate the chambers of the heart; one (or more) of the valves doesn't open enough to allow blood to flow freely (stenosis) or doesn't close tightly enough to prevent blood from flowing backward (regurgitation). Stenosis and/or regurgitation can develop in any of the four valves, but both are more common on the left side of the heart involving the aortic or mitral valves. Certain forms of valve disease are related to advanced age, but others may be related to infections or other conditions.

Conditions Related to the Circulatory System

STROKE AND CEREBROVASCULAR DISEASE

Stroke (cerebrovascular accident) is to the brain what a heart attack is to the heart, and it usually happens for the same reason: when blood flow is blocked or interrupted. When any part of the brain is deprived of nutrient-rich blood, irreversible damage can be the result. This is why, as with symptoms of heart attack, it is important to get stroke victims treated as soon as possible. Symptoms of a stroke include speech abnormalities, facial drooping, and arm or leg weakness.

PERIPHERAL VASCULAR DISEASE

Peripheral artery disease (PAD) is a disease in the arteries far from the heart. PAD results from atherosclerosis (the formation of fatty deposits in the blood vessels), which prevents sufficient flow of blood to the kidneys, arms, legs, and feet. Its consequences can be anything from cramping of the legs, either when walking or resting, to permanent damage to these body parts if blood is severely restricted. If the kidneys are involved, chronic kidney disease or kidney failure can be the result. People with PAD are also at a very high risk of having a stroke or a heart attack.

Deep vein thrombosis is a serious condition where blood clots form in the veins, usually in the leg. These clots can dislodge, travel through the bloodstream to an artery in a lung, and block blood flow, resulting in a condition called *pulmonary embolism* (see below).

HYPERTENSION / HYPERTENSIVE HEART DISEASE

Hypertension, or high blood pressure, is a common condition that usually causes no symptoms but, when undiagnosed or untreated, can lead to heart attack, heart failure, stroke, kidney disease, and even vision loss. Hypertension can be easily diagnosed and kept under control with regular checkups and lifestyle choices, including managing weight, increasing activity, and healthy food choices. For some, medication is also needed. Hypertension is more prevalent in postmenopausal women and even more common in Black women.

Hypertensive heart disease refers to heart damage that results from long-standing undiagnosed or inadequately treated high blood pressure; it may lead to coronary artery disease, heart failure, and thickening of the heart muscle.

OTHER

Pulmonary embolism is a sudden blockage in an artery going to the lung caused by a blood clot that was formed someplace else in the body. This blood clot is capable of causing permanent damage to the lung, and this can prevent other organs from getting the oxygenated blood they need to function. A pulmonary embolism can lead to heart failure or death, whether caused by one large clot or many smaller clots.

Begin to Identify Your Risk Factors for Heart Disease

We've discussed earlier that ischemic heart disease describes the full range of coronary artery disease (CAD). Because this is the most common form of heart disease, it's important to spend a bit more time understanding how it occurs and identifying your risk factors. Ischemic heart disease begins with damage to the lining and inner layers of the coronary arteries. Surprisingly, this damage to the lining of the arteries can begin as early as young adulthood and lead to a buildup of plaque in the coronary arteries that continues throughout adulthood. Over time, this plaque can slowly grow to narrow or completely obstruct the artery, resulting in the chest pain or discomfort that we call angina. In the case of a nonobstructing plaque, the plaque can acutely rupture, leading to a heart attack. This is called a *vulnerable plaque*. Even if it doesn't rupture, this hardened plaque builds up inside the coronary arteries, causing them to narrow, and this reduces the flow of oxygen-rich blood to the heart muscle.

But what does this mean for you, and which are the risk factors that have been shown to increase your chances of suffering damage to these arteries?

To help you begin to think critically about your risk factors, we have separated them into three categories: modifiable risk factors (those that can be treated to lessen the risk), nonmodifiable risk factors (those that are important to know but cannot be changed), and risk factors that are unique to women. In the next chapter, we'll examine in greater detail each of these risk factors, but for now, use the box below to identify the specific risk factors that are of concern to you. These will help you begin to build a better understanding of areas that you can target to develop a healthier heart.

NONMODIFIABLE RISK FACTORS

- ☐ Heredity (including family history, race, and ethnicity)
- ☐ Age
- ☐ Gender

MODIFIABLE RISK FACTORS

- ☐ Smoking, including secondhand smoke
- ☐ High blood pressure (hypertension)
- ☐ Abnormal blood sugar (diabetes or prediabetes)
- ☐ Elevated cholesterol (hyperlipidemia)
- ☐ Sedentary lifestyle
- ☐ Being overweight or obese

RISK FACTORS THAT ARE UNIQUE TO WOMEN

- ☐ Pregnancy-related hypertension (eclampsia or pre-eclampsia) or abnormalities of sugar (gestational diabetes)
- ☐ Other APOs (adverse pregnancy outcomes), including low-birth-weight babies
- ☐ Other gynecologic events—age at first period, early menopause, polycystic ovary disease, even choice of birth control

OTHER CONTRIBUTING FACTORS

- ☐ Stress
- ☐ Insufficient sleep
- ☐ Substance abuse disorder
- ☐ Poor diet and nutrition
- ☐ Autoimmune disease such as lupus or rheumatoid arthritis
- ☐ Chronic kidney disease
- ☐ Depression, anxiety, and other psychosocial risk factors

You now have a better understanding of the key features of the heart and how heart disease affects how the heart works. Keep this chapter handy; as you read through the chapters that follow, you may find it helpful to turn back to these definitions—or the model of the heart—to deepen your knowledge. But next, let's turn our attention to how best to prevent and control these risk factors so you can live a heart-healthier life. As you read on, you'll find the tools you need to identify your personal risk of developing CAD, minimize the impact those risk factors may have on your life, and start your journey to living a heart-smart life!

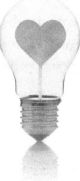

Chapter Three

ASSESSING YOUR RISK FOR HEART DISEASE

Our goal in this book is to equip you with the knowledge and tools you'll need to live a heart-smart, heart-healthy life and to get you started with a six-week plan. Each day, you have the opportunity to make choices that will protect you from the likelihood of developing heart disease. Every day, women across the country are learning how to make healthy, permanent changes to their lives in order to prevent heart disease or lessen its impact.

Rebecca

In chapter 1, we introduced you to Rebecca, a forty-two-year-old White woman. We now want to share with you more of Rebecca's story and her journey to a healthier heart.

For twenty years, Rebecca has worked as a nurse on the cardiac service at a large hospital. But one day she found herself in the waiting room of the imaging center of that hospital not as a nurse but as a patient scheduled for a stress test. As she waited for her name to be called, she reflected on the sequence of events that led her here.

It had all started the previous month, when she began feeling fatigued and had difficulty catching her breath when she climbed stairs or walked quickly when food shopping. For the past three years, she had been going through the stress of a divorce after finding out her husband had been unfaithful. Now that her divorce was finalized, she was finally feeling optimistic about the future. But Rebecca didn't know how to slow down and take it easy. She typically worked four ten-hour shifts each week, with most of that time spent on her feet. In addition, she had a busy domestic life with two teenagers at home—a son in high school and a daughter in community college—and she also cared for her increasingly disabled mother. Rebecca often found herself unable to get a good night's sleep.

Ironically, Rebecca's job as a nurse was to care for women and men recovering from heart attacks, yet not for one moment did she consider that her own symptoms of fatigue and shortness of breath were warning signs of heart disease. She had no chest pain and she was still able to do her job, so her symptoms could not possibly have meant that she had heart disease.

In the waiting room, nervously waiting to be called in for her stress test, she distracted herself by picking up a brochure that described the symptoms of heart disease in women and how they can differ from the typical male symptoms. What she read made the hairs on the back of her neck stand up. She realized that she, a healthcare professional, didn't even know that the warning signs of heart disease in women might be different from those in men!

Rebecca thought about her constant exhaustion and recalled those occasions when she experienced mild upper back pain—usually when climbing stairs—that she ignored or attributed to a number of excuses: weight gain, lack of regular physical activity, the stress related to her divorce, and being a single mom and caregiver.

But as she continued to read, she began to acknowledge the fact that she had many of the risk factors for heart disease, including:

- Early menopause (hers began at age forty)

- Treatment for mild hypertension

- Slow but steady weight gain to nearly obese (mostly stored around a thirty-nine-inch waist)

- High body mass index (BMI), of 29

In addition, Rebecca recalled that the bloodwork done at her yearly visit to her internist six months ago showed she was prediabetic and at risk for diabetes, and her blood pressure was high. At that time, her doctor had put her on an antihypertensive medication and reassured her that if she made some changes to her diet and decreased her waist circumference, she would be in good shape. They agreed to revisit this at her next appointment.

Rebecca had the classic signs, but she hadn't put them together, and initially, neither had her doctor. And here she was, scheduled for a stress test only because of the urging of a worried colleague.

One week earlier, at the end of a ten-hour shift, Rebecca had experienced left-upper-back pain. She felt extremely fatigued and was short of breath. Her colleague noticed her sitting and resting before being able to head home and convinced her to speak to the cardiologist on call that night. The cardiologist wisely suggested that she be evaluated to find out why she was feeling this way.

As she sat in the waiting room, knowing what she now knew, Rebecca was concerned. She was keeping her fingers crossed that she would be fine.

Rebecca's wake-up call came just in time. Her stress test revealed that she didn't have significant ischemic heart disease; her symptoms were caused by poorly controlled hypertension. In fact, her blood pressure at the end of her stress test was markedly elevated, at 210/110. She realized that while she was taking the blood pressure medication prescribed by her doctor, she had never followed up with him to check to be sure that it was effective and that the dosage was correct.

At her follow-up visit a few days later, her cardiologist customized the same Six S.T.E.P.S. in Six Weeks Program you will find in part two of this book. Rebecca's progress was impressive. By her next visit to her cardiologist, she had lost seven pounds and one inch off her waist, her blood pressure was within normal range at 118/78, she was sleeping better, and she had more energy.

A Reminder of Why This Matters

Rebecca's progress demonstrates that heart health knowledge matters—and that a healthier heart is possible. Remember the key statistics we discussed at the start of this book:

- One woman dies every eighty seconds from cardiovascular disease.

- One in every three deaths of women each year is caused by cardiovascular disease.

- Ninety percent of women have one or more risk factors for cardiovascular disease.

- Fewer women survive their first year after a heart attack than men.

- Certain risk factors for heart disease are more potent for Black, Latina, and South Asian women.

But there is good news in the midst of these sober statistics. Our goal in this book is to equip you to have your own success story, just like Rebecca. We know from the findings of the American Heart Association, through their Go Red for Women movement, that[5]:

- 80 percent of heart disease is preventable through lifestyle changes and education.

- Women who participate in heart-healthy programs actually do reap the benefits they promise by adopting healthier habits.

- Over the past ten years, the death rate of women from heart disease has decreased more than 30 percent, and one of the key components to this is improved awareness and knowledge about lowering our risk for developing heart disease.

These encouraging statistics are the direct result of an increased understanding on the part of the medical community about how women present with heart disease as well as the healthy behavioral changes women have made. These changes include such things as maintaining a healthy weight; moving more; making healthy diet changes; keeping track of cholesterol, blood sugar, and blood pressure levels; and partnering with their doctors to learn how to start and optimize a heart-health plan.

HEART HEALTH KNOWLEDGE MATTERS—AND A HEALTHIER HEART IS POSSIBLE.

---

5   "Preventing Cardiovascular Disease," Go Red for Women, accessed November 16, 2021, https://www.goredforwomen.org/en/about-heart-disease-in-women/preventing-cardiovascular-disease.

It's possible to improve your heart's health. Taking an active role in your health will help you feel better and live longer.

Make It Personal: Take Stock of Your Risk Factors

When it comes to risk factors for heart disease, the science is clear: the sooner you identify and address your risk factors, the less likely you are to develop heart disease and the healthier you will be. We hope you'll take the following, literally, to heart.

Although women generally have the same heart disease risk factors as men, there are some risk factors that either affect women exclusively, such as pregnancy-related issues and issues surrounding menopause, or affect women differently—for example, diabetes, which raises the risk of heart disease more in women than in men. What is common to both sexes is that our risk for heart disease and heart attack rises with the number of risk factors each of us has, as well as the severity of each of those risk factors. What's more, risk factors tend to "snowball" and worsen each other's effects, and sometimes, having one risk factor increases the likelihood that you will have another. For example, being overweight or obese raises the chances of your also having hypertension or prediabetes. Complicating this snowball effect is that some risk factors are worse than others. For example, smoking and diabetes put you at far greater risk for heart disease and heart attack than other risk factors.

It is important to remember that:

- 90 percent of women have one or more risk factors for developing heart disease.[6]

---

6   "Causes and Prevention of Heart Disease," Go Red for Women, accessed November 16, 2021, https://www.goredforwomen.org/en/about-heart-disease-in-women/facts/causes-and-prevention-of-heart-disease.

- Women also are at greater risk than men when it comes to having heart disease or a stroke, especially if they are Black, Latina, or of South Asian descent.

But there is a way to significantly improve those odds by making simple lifestyle changes. For example, sustained moderate exercise can significantly decrease your chance of heart disease by positively impacting several risk factors, such as lowering blood pressure, improving cholesterol levels, and achieving a healthy weight.

Identify, Address, and Modify Your Risk Factors

The goal of this book is to empower you to identify, address, and modify the factors that put you at risk for heart disease. As medical professionals, we fully recognize that some of the most potent risk factors are the most difficult to address. Quitting smoking, losing weight, managing stress, and becoming more active may seem overwhelming at first. But we will offer you suggestions, advice, and tips on how to start the process toward living a heart-smarter life. This is not an all-or-nothing proposition! Each small change can make a difference and have a big impact on your heart health.

It's also important to note that this should not be a solo effort. If you haven't identified a primary care physician who understands issues related to women's heart health, you will find suggestions in Week 4 of the Six S.T.E.P.S. in Six Weeks Program on how to choose a doctor with whom you can partner. If you are already seeing a doctor or are taking medications for other risk factors, then be sure to follow your doctor's instructions regarding lifestyle choices and take your medication exactly as prescribed. Don't be shy about asking questions if there is something you don't understand. If you're diabetic, be diligent about checking your blood sugar and keeping your numbers in the normal range. There are dozens of small decisions we make each day that give us the opportunity to improve our heart health and minimize our chances of ever having a heart attack.

Create a Personal Health Inventory

As a first step on your journey to a healthier heart, you will need an accurate inventory of your overall health. Keeping this inventory will be one of the biggest assets in your quest to stay heart healthy. A physician or nurse makes notes in your chart when you come in for an office visit, and you need to do the same for yourself. This is the start of your journal, which we call your "Personal Health Inventory." Keeping track of all the details about your personal health in one document will be a real eye-opener. This information will help you keep track of the things you want to discuss with your doctor and serve as a foundation to allow you and your doctor to customize an overall health plan. It also will be a way to have all of your health information at your fingertips, including your family medical history, your personal medical history (all surgeries, medical procedures, hospitalizations, pregnancy-related issues, etc.), allergies, the medications or supplements you currently take and their dosage (including any reactions or side effects experienced from other medications you have previously taken), your insurance numbers, your doctor's instructions, and your treatment plan.

A journal can take whatever form you prefer. It will be a constantly evolving record, and it will be important to keep it up to date. Some people like to use a fancy notebook, while others use an electronic tablet or smartphone, a legal pad, or even a three-ring binder. Whatever works best for you is all that matters, but if you opt for keeping a digital journal, be sure to secure and protect all data appropriately and optimize privacy settings.

At the end of this chapter, you'll find a template for your Personal Health Inventory. As you read through the remainder of this chapter, you may wish to make some notes now to begin to create this personal resource, starting with the following.

Risk Factors You Cannot Change

FAMILY HISTORY AND GENETICS

The most important risk factor that you cannot change is your family history. We are all products of our family's genetic makeup, and our risk of heart disease is greatly impacted by our genetic composition. Think of your family members, take stock of their health, and make a list of any medical issues they have. Start with your immediate family. For example, do you have a male parent or sibling, living or dead, who had a heart attack or stroke or suffered from heart disease at age fifty-five or younger or a female parent or sibling who had the same at age sixty-five or younger? If so, write down his or her relationship to you and as detailed a description as you can provide of the nature of his or her heart condition.

Having parents or siblings with early heart disease increases your risk too. Your Personal Health Inventory will show you if you are at risk through heredity. Discussing your family history of heart disease accurately with your doctor is an excellent first step to early identification, proper screening, and treatment for you.

Even though a family history of heart disease significantly increases your risk, knowing about it can make all the difference in your own health. Once you are aware that you may be at high risk, you have the information that will allow you to make changes. In certain circumstances, more aggressive risk factor identification and modification may be appropriate for those with a family history of premature heart disease.

It is useful to note in your Inventory other important health conditions of your immediate family.

RACE AND ETHNICITY

The past two decades of medical and scientific research have shown us the importance of studying heart disease in gender-, race-, and ethnicity-specific ways. Just as we learned that heart disease in women can be different from heart disease in men, we have also learned that Black, Latina, and South Asian women may be affected by risk factors differently than White women. Black and Hispanic women are generally at higher risk due to the prevalence and potency of such risk factors as high blood pressure, diabetes, physical inactivity, and challenges with maintaining a healthy weight. Women of South Asian descent are more likely to have abnormal cholesterol and triglycerides and prediabetes profiles, which in turn increase the likelihood of having heart disease. Simply being aware of these additional risks and how they are influenced by your heritage will give you a head start in preventing potential health problems or treating current ones.

Our goal is to educate all women so that they can narrow the odds of developing heart disease and learn about the additional health problems that some of us carry in our genes. Because of genetic factors, you might be at higher risk than someone in another racial or ethnic group, but the playing field is leveled when it comes to environmental factors—if you know what to do. The key is prevention, and the Six S.T.E.P.S. in Six Weeks Program is designed to help you get there.

Note your race and ethnic background in your Personal Health Inventory so that you can discuss with your physician whether your race or ethnicity brings with it any additional risks or requires any special precautions on your road to heart health.

AGE

The risk of developing heart disease increases with age. In addition, postmenopausal women are at greater risk than premenopausal women. So make a note of your present age in your Personal Health Inventory and, if applicable, the age you went through menopause.

Risk Factors You Can Modify

DIABETES (HIGH BLOOD SUGAR) AND PREDIABETES

Diabetes is a disease in which the body's blood sugar level is too high. This is because the body doesn't make insulin (generally referred to as type 1 diabetes) or does make insulin but doesn't process it effectively (generally referred to as type 2 diabetes). Insulin is a hormone that helps move blood sugar into cells where it's used for energy. Over time, a high blood sugar level is dangerous because it contributes to increased plaque buildup in the arteries. Diabetes and prediabetes raise the risk of heart disease more in women than in men, and having diabetes can almost double a woman's risk of developing heart disease. Prediabetes is a condition in which the blood sugar level is higher than normal but not as high as with diabetes. However, prediabetes also puts you at higher risk for developing both diabetes and heart disease.

Before menopause, estrogen provides women some protection against heart disease, but women who are diabetic lose the protective effects of estrogen. Uncontrolled diabetes is a particularly worrisome risk factor for women but becomes even more dangerous for women who have other, simultaneous risk factors such as high cholesterol, hypertension, or obesity. If you have diabetes, prediabetes, or insulin resistance, add this fact to your Personal Health Inventory.

If you have diabetes, it is very important that you check your blood regularly, make smart food choices, maintain an ideal body weight, and exercise regularly. If you are taking oral medication or using insulin, use as directed. People who learn to manage their diabetes can live long, healthy, and active lives.

The blood test to diagnose diabetes and prediabetes is the hemoglobin A1c (HbA1c). It provides clinicians with an accurate picture of what a person's average blood sugar levels have been over a period of weeks/months.

Normal HbA1c:	under 5.7 percent
Prediabetes:	5.7 to 6.4 percent
Diabetes:	6.5 percent or above confirmed on two separate occasions

Recently, the medical community recommended that this test be the primary test used to diagnose all forms of diabetes, as opposed to the fasting blood glucose test of years past. Testing for diabetes during pregnancy (known as gestational diabetes) is defined according to a different protocol, something called a "glucose challenge test."

HYPERTENSION (HIGH BLOOD PRESSURE)

Blood pressure is the measured force of the blood against the artery walls. This pressure is recorded in two numbers. The higher number is the systolic blood pressure, which represents the pressure in the arteries when the heart is pumping blood, and the lower number is the diastolic blood pressure, which represents the pressure in the arteries when the heart muscle is relaxing (i.e., between heartbeats).

In 2017, the American Heart Association updated their blood pressure guidelines. The chart below reflects these guidelines and the categories established by the American Heart Association with respect to hypertension:

BLOOD PRESSURE CATEGORY	SYSTOLIC mm Hg (upper number)		DIASTOLIC mm Hg (lower number)
Normal	Less than 120	and	Less than 80
Elevated	120-129	and	Less than 80
High Blood Pressure (Hypertension) Stage 1	130-139	or	80-89
High Blood Pressure (Hypertension) Stage 2	140 or Higher	or	90 or Higher
Hypertensive Crisis (consult your doctor immediately)	Higher than 180	and/or	Higher than 120

When a person has high blood pressure, the heart muscle works harder than it should, which can lead to atherosclerosis and other heart problems such as heart failure. There are no real symptoms of high blood pressure, so if you haven't visited your doctor in some time, you may not know that you have it. It is very important to have it checked regularly. According to the American Heart Association, prevalence of hypertension (HTN) significantly increases with age, with over 65 percent of women older than sixty-five years having HTN.[7]

Again, we want you to think about your relatives, as high blood pressure often runs in families. Make a note of any who suffer from it in your Personal Health Inventory. Additionally, high blood pressure often affects women who are overweight and/or eat a diet high in salt. If you have been diagnosed with high blood pressure, including gestational hypertension (even if it resolved after giving birth), note that as well.

LIPIDS (LDL AND HDL CHOLESTEROL AND TRIGLYCERIDES)

In recent years, our understanding of the impact of elevated cholesterol on our health has been significantly improved. Explaining cholesterol can be confusing, but we can simplify it. Cholesterol is a soft, fatlike substance found in the cells of the body and circulating in the blood. If you have too much cholesterol, it interacts with other substances to form plaque in the lining of the arteries, causing atherosclerosis.

Cholesterol travels in the bloodstream in small packages called lipoproteins. The two major kinds of lipoproteins are *low-density-lipoprotein (LDL)* cholesterol and *high-density-lipoprotein (HDL)* cholesterol. LDL cholesterol is sometimes called "bad" cholesterol because it carries cholesterol to tissues, including heart arteries, while HDL cholesterol is sometimes called "good" cholesterol because it helps remove cholesterol from the heart arteries.

---

7   "AHA Prevention Guidelines," *Hypertension* 75 (2020): 1334–57, doi: 10.1161/
     HYPERTENSIONAHA.120.15026.

A blood test called a lipid panel is used to measure cholesterol levels. This test gives information about total cholesterol, LDL cholesterol, HDL cholesterol, and triglycerides, another type of fat found in the blood, which we will discuss in more detail below.

Cholesterol levels are measured in milligrams (mg) of cholesterol per deciliter (dL) of blood. An abnormal cholesterol panel is generally defined as total cholesterol of greater than 200 mg/dL, with an LDL cholesterol level greater than 100 mg/dL, and/or an HDL cholesterol level less than 50 mg/dL.

In addition to cholesterol, there are *triglycerides*, which represent the most common type of fat in the body. Too much presents a powerful risk factor for women. We now know that a woman's HDL cholesterol and triglyceride levels predict her risk for CHD better than her total cholesterol or LDL cholesterol levels. A triglyceride level greater than or equal to 150 mg/dL is considered elevated.

The American Heart Association and the American College of Cardiology have created a more personalized approach to identifying your risk for heart disease, called the ASCVD (AtheroSclerotic CardioVascular Disease) Risk Estimator. Women who have not previously had a heart attack or stroke can use this tool. It uses your information (including race, gender, age, cholesterol numbers, and blood pressure) to calculate your risk of heart disease. You can find the ASCVD tool at the American College of Cardiology's website (acc.org) or download the app from iTunes or Google Play.

If you or an immediate family member has high cholesterol or triglyceride levels, please note this in your Personal Health Inventory.

Exercise and a healthy diet low in sugar and saturated fats help decrease cholesterol levels. There is also evidence that cholesterol-lowering medications, called statins, can reduce the incidence of heart disease and heart attack for women.

OVERWEIGHT/OBESITY

People who are overweight have a greater chance of also having high blood pressure, diabetes, and elevated cholesterol levels. An overweight or obese woman is three times more likely to have heart disease than a woman of normal body weight for her height. Being overweight is a very common problem today among all women, as are the health issues it creates.

The interesting thing about weight loss is that, for many, just losing as little as five to eight pounds can help to get blood pressure under control, improve blood sugar, and decrease lipid levels, thereby lowering the risk of developing heart disease or having a heart attack. Even women who continue to carry their "baby weight" in the first year after giving birth have been shown to be at higher cardiovascular risk.

What's important for you to understand is the fact that it's not just how much extra weight you carry but *where* you carry it. Women who carry much of their fat around the waist are referred to as apple-shaped and are at highest risk for heart disease. Women who carry most of their fat on their hips and thighs are referred to as pear-shaped and are at lower risk for heart disease than those who are apple-shaped.

To get the full picture of how excess weight affects your risk, you need to know your body mass index (BMI) and waist measurement. The BMI is the measure of an individual's body fat based on his or her weight in relation to her height. If you have a BMI greater than 24.9 and a waist measurement greater than thirty-five inches, you're at increased risk. If your waist measurement divided by your hip measurement is greater than 0.9, you're also at increased risk.

> IT'S NOT JUST HOW MUCH EXTRA WEIGHT YOU CARRY BUT *WHERE* YOU CARRY IT.

CALCULATE YOUR BMI

A simple formula will help you calculate your body mass index (BMI):

Your weight (in pounds)

÷

your height (in inches) squared

×

703.

For example, if you weigh 150 pounds and you are 5'5" (or 65 inches), the formula would be

150 ÷ (65 × 65) × 703 = 24.96.

According to the National Heart, Lung, and Blood Institute (NHLBI), you can interpret your BMI in this way:[8]

- Underweight = less than 18.5

- Healthy weight = 18.5–24.9

- Overweight = 25–29.9

- Obesity = BMI of 30 or higher

If you prefer not to do the math yourself, you can find a BMI calculator on the NHLBI website (www.nhlbi.nih.gov); you can also download an app for your smartphone.

---

8   "Calculate Your Body Mass Index," National Heart, Lung, and Blood Institute," accessed November 16, 2021, https://www.nhlbi.nih.gov/health/educational/lose_ wt/BMI/bmicalc.htm.

METABOLIC SYNDROME

The term *metabolic syndrome* refers to a group of risk factors that tend to occur together. These include low HDL, high triglycerides, elevated blood pressure, abnormal blood sugar, and abdominal obesity. A diagnosis of metabolic syndrome is made if you have three of these five risk factors.

CIGARETTE SMOKING / SECONDHAND SMOKE

Not only does smoking increase the risk of having heart disease and a heart attack, but it is the leading preventable cause of heart disease. Just in case you need a little more persuading, women smokers are six times more likely to have coronary artery disease than nonsmokers. Smoking has a negative impact on cholesterol levels, as there is evidence that it encourages blood platelets to clump within coronary arteries, making a heart attack more likely. Smoking also has an impact on microvascular dysfunction, leading to blood vessels that do not behave normally, with resulting angina and heart attack (see chapter 2).

Smoking only a few cigarettes a day can *double* your risk of coronary artery disease as compared to a nonsmoker, and we're not even mentioning lung cancer, COPD, macular degeneration, and a host of other problems that smoking complicates, such as diabetes and high blood pressure. The good news is that when you quit smoking that risk starts decreasing immediately, and over time the risk goes away.

Exposure to secondhand smoke increases the risk of heart disease in the same way. So ask your smoking friends and relatives to step outside if they want to smoke and you want to stay healthy.

If you still smoke or live in a household where smoking is tolerated, then note that in your Personal Health Inventory and work with your housemates or family members to develop a plan to create a smoke-free living environment.

Recently, some people have tried to cut back on their cigarette smoking by turning to e-cigarettes or "vaping." However, clinical studies on the effects of e-cigarettes suggest that toxic effects of nicotine in traditional cigarettes also exist with e-cigarettes. At this time, we do not recommend the use of e-cigarettes as a tool to stop smoking.

There is no way to sugarcoat this message: smoking kills. There are many new medications and quitting aids on the market (with and without a prescription) that can help you kick the habit. Schedule a visit with your doctor and discuss the best way to stop. You can also get help by calling the National Cancer Institute's Smoking Quit Line (1-877-44U-Quit) for advice provided by their trained personnel or by contacting your local hospital or health system; many have smoking cessation programs for community members. With the current price of cigarettes, quitting will also save you money. So quit today and start saving for that vacation, that special dress, or that show you've been wanting to see. What a great way to celebrate your new, healthier lifestyle.

PHYSICAL INACTIVITY

You've heard it many times before: it's important to be active. Please understand: our message here is to empower you! We're not saying that you need to join a gym, hire a trainer, or spend hours daily working out, but we are saying that to keep your heart healthy, you must maintain an active lifestyle. The good news is that small steps will make a big difference. Changes as minor as adding a brisk walk for thirty minutes each day (three ten-minute walks have the same benefit), taking the stairs instead of the elevator, or parking your car at the far end of the shopping center lot all contribute to a more active you! The advice is simple: we all need to "choose to move" more.

An inactive lifestyle leads to a higher incidence of high blood pressure, obesity, and elevated cholesterol. According to the National Cancer Institute, higher levels of physical activity are also linked to lowered risks of certain types of cancer, including breast cancer, bladder cancer, colon cancer, and endometrial cancer.[9]

You may have heard the term *exercise-related cardioprotection*. This refers to the fact that physical activity leads to improvement in many of the risk factors described previously. Active women have a significantly decreased incidence of heart disease. If you are not moving around as much as you should, add this risk factor to your Personal Health Inventory. Remember, too, that any movement is good. This includes cleaning the house, walking the dog, running around after the kids or grandkids, dancing, bicycling, etc. Thirty to forty-five minutes of activity three times a week is all you need for a healthy heart and a more fit you.

A wearable tracking device can be useful for counting your steps as well as reminding you to get up and walk around if you have been sitting for longer than one hour. Read more about these devices in Week 2 of our Six S.T.E.P.S. in Six Weeks Program.

STRESS

Stress is something we must all learn to live with, but too much stress takes its toll on our heart health. How we react to stress varies from person to person, but most of us could benefit from finding creative ways to make our lives less stressful. We've all been there—some things may roll off our

9   "Physical Activity and Cancer," National Cancer Institute, accessed November 16, 2021, https://www.cancer.gov/about-cancer/causes-prevention/risk/obesity/physical-activity-fact-sheet.

backs today but send us into a tailspin tomorrow. And we all have friends who seem to manage stress beautifully, while others simply do not.

There are also different types of stress. Events over which we have no control may wreak havoc on our lives when we least expect it, but sometimes we experience stress that we have created ourselves.

Here's an example: If you are the type of person who leaves everything to the last minute, you may then experience anxiety trying to meet a deadline or be on time. But you can implement some time-management lifestyle changes to make your life run more smoothly. Or maybe you stress out and feel guilty about taking time out for yourself to relax. But having no downtime takes its toll on your health. So if you are feeling stressed for *any* reason, make a note of it in your Personal Health Inventory, along with your reasons for feeling this way.

Learning how to manage stress is important for overall health as well as heart health. Take a look at your daily routine, including your personal, family, and work relationships, with an eye to lessening stress.

SLEEP

Not getting enough sleep can set you up for heart problems. Without adequate sleep, the body simply cannot function as it should. Our circadian rhythm (a cycle of approximately twenty-four hours) tells our bodies when to sleep, rise, and eat. If you don't have regular sleep habits or don't get enough sleep, your body's functions will not be in balance. When you stay awake for too long, you are fighting the body's natural tendency to rest, and that can be harmful to your overall health.

Chronically disrupted or insufficient sleep can affect everything from your critical thinking ability to your mental health and sex drive. Lack of sleep may actually even increase your risk of death from all causes. If you rely on taking medication to control important health issues like high blood pressure, then the efficacy of the medications may be lessened by poor sleep habits.

The bottom line is that your body needs rest to recharge itself, to keep the immune system in peak condition, and to keep your circadian rhythm in its normal cycle. We all need enough sleep to ensure that we stay healthy and safe, make sound decisions, and can adequately deal with the stresses and challenges of daily life.

Seven hours of sleep every night is the minimum amount of sleep we need. Sleep time cannot be "made up" on weekends! If you are unable to get enough sleep, note it in your Personal Health Inventory; it can be an important clue if you develop health issues, start forgetting things, or just don't feel like yourself.

Getting adequate rest is one of the most important things you can do for your overall health and well-being. If you are well rested, you'll feel more alert, you'll have the energy needed to exercise, you'll look better, and you'll be better able to fight off illness.

Risk Factors That Are Unique to or More Potent for Women

AUTOIMMUNE DISEASES

Recent research shows that in women the presence of autoimmune diseases such as lupus and rheumatoid arthritis has been linked to a higher risk of atherosclerosis, which, as you will recall from chapter 2, is the buildup of plaque and fat in the arteries. Plaque buildup in the coronary arteries can lead to blockages in blood flow to the heart, which can result in heart attack. Women suffer from autoimmune diseases at a significantly higher rate than men. If you suffer from an autoimmune disease such as lupus or rheumatoid arthritis and have other risk factors for heart disease, you are at greater risk for developing heart disease at a younger age. This autoimmune condition also inhibits the natural protection of estrogen in premenopausal women.

The human body's immune system functions as a complex network of special cells and organs designed to defend the body against germs and other foreign invaders. At its core, your immune system has the unique ability to identify your own tissues and distinguish them from foreign invaders like bacteria or viruses. But sometimes a flaw develops that hinders its ability to make this distinction, and the body starts producing autoantibodies that attack normal cells by mistake. Special cells called regulatory T cells, whose job it is to keep the immune system in line, also fail. The end result is a misguided attack on the body by itself.

Which parts of the body are affected depends on which of the eighty known types of autoimmune diseases is at work. Although there are no cures for these autoimmune diseases, treatment options have been continually improving. In addition to medications, a healthy weight, physical activity, and sufficient sleep have all been shown to have a positive effect on symptoms. Autoimmune diseases seem to run in families, so be sure to include information in your Personal Health Inventory about any family members with any of these conditions.

Rheumatoid Arthritis

Rheumatoid arthritis, also known as RA, is the most common type of autoimmune disease and is more common among women than men. It tends to strike women at younger ages than men, and women tend to respond less well to treatment. The disease attacks the lining of the joints throughout the body, making them painful, stiff, swollen, and deformed.

Systemic Lupus Erythematosus

Systemic lupus erythematosus, also known as SLE, is the most common type of lupus and the type of the disease that attacks connective tissue. It mainly affects women, but men do get it. Lupus can produce painful and swollen joints as well as harm the heart, kidneys, skin, lungs, and other organs. The disease does not have a predictable course; women with lupus are subject to flare-ups followed by remission.

Some signs of lupus include:

- "Butterfly" rash across the nose and cheeks

- Rashes on other parts of the body

- Painful or swollen joints and muscle pain

- Hair loss

- Headaches and severe fatigue

Sjögren's Syndrome

Sjögren's (SHOH-grins) syndrome is a disorder of the immune system that targets the glands that make moisture. Its most common symptoms are dry eyes and dry mouth. Sjögren's syndrome is often seen in those who have other immune system disorders such as rheumatoid arthritis and lupus. Women are affected more often than men, and it is more prevalent in those over forty.

Symptoms can include:

- Dry, burning, or itchy eyes, nose, and mouth (with increased dental decay)

- Vaginal dryness

- Sore or cracked tongue and dry or peeling lips

- Dry or burning feeling in throat

- Difficulty talking, chewing, or swallowing

- Dry skin or rash

- Joint pain, stiffness or swelling

- Fatigue

Antiphospholipid Syndrome

In antiphospholipid syndrome, the immune system mistakenly attacks proteins in the blood, causing blood clots to form within arteries or veins of the kidneys, lungs, or brain, which may cause deep vein thrombosis, a stroke, heart attack, or pulmonary embolism, depending on the location of the clot. It is often the clinical explanation for repeated miscarriage. There is no cure, but medications can reduce the risk of blood clots.

PREGNANCY-RELATED RISK FACTORS

Women who experience certain pregnancy-related complications are at an increased risk for heart disease. These are referred to as "adverse pregnancy outcomes."

Some of these risk factors include the following:

Gestational Diabetes

Pregnant women who develop elevated blood sugar that first appears during pregnancy are said to have gestational diabetes. Generally, gestational diabetes resolves after delivery. However, women who have had gestational diabetes have a significantly higher risk of developing diabetes within five to ten years after delivery and a higher lifetime risk for heart disease.

Gestational Hypertension

This is high blood pressure that develops after week twenty of pregnancy but resolves after delivery.

Preeclampsia

This is a serious condition of pregnancy characterized by high blood pressure and sometimes elevated protein in the urine. It usually develops after week twenty of pregnancy but can be diagnosed even after delivery. Preeclampsia can lead to serious complications if not treated in a timely manner. Women with diabetes and obesity before pregnancy are at an increased risk of developing preeclampsia. Although typically the symptoms go away after delivery, women who have experienced preeclampsia have an increased risk of developing high blood pressure later in life. Women who had preeclampsia during pregnancy have a four times greater risk for heart disease.[10]

Eclampsia

This is a rare and severe complication of preeclampsia in which there are seizures resulting in periods of disturbed brain activity that can cause episodes of staring, decreased alertness, and violent shaking (convulsions). Eclampsia affects about one in every two hundred women with preeclampsia.

Gestational diabetes, gestational hypertension, preeclampsia, and eclampsia are all linked to an increased lifetime risk of heart disease, including coronary artery disease, heart attack, and heart failure. It is important to tell your doctor if you had any of these conditions so your heart disease risk can be accurately assessed.

---

10   "Pregnancy complications linked to heightened risk of heart disease and stroke in later life," BMJ, July 10, 2020, https://www.bmj.com/company/newsroom/pregnancy-complications-linked-to-heightened-risk-of-heart-disease-and-stroke-in-later-life/.

OTHER REPRODUCTIVE HEALTH RISK FACTORS

In addition to pregnancy-related risk factors for heart disease, other elements of your reproductive health may impact your heart health.

A team of UK researchers has found that several factors may increase your risk for heart disease:[11]

- Starting your period early (before age twelve)

- Diagnosis of polycystic ovary syndrome—a condition that causes hormonal imbalances and metabolic issues

- Experiencing a miscarriage or stillbirth

- Early menopause (before age forty)

- Preterm delivery

These are all factors that should be included in your Personal Health Inventory. On the pages that follow, we've supplied a template that you can complete and use as a valuable resource for informed conversations with your health provider. But this is only one possible format. You may find it more helpful to track this data on your laptop or smartphone or to log this information in a notebook or journal. What's most important is that you find the system that works for you and get started!

---

11   Ibid.

MY PERSONAL HEALTH INVENTORY

Use this space to note key information about your health and your family's health history.

My birth date: _____

My race: _____

My ethnicity: _____

My medical history (pregnancies, surgeries, procedures, and hospitalizations as well as chronic conditions): _____

_____

_____

_____

Allergies: _____

_____

_____

_____

Current medications and vitamins/supplements (including dosage and frequency): _____

_____

_____

_____

Previous regimens of medication, vitamins/supplements, and all other over-the-counter products (including any reactions or side effects): _____

_____

_____

_____

My height: _____

My weight: _____

My BMI: _____

My family members with specific health issues and the age of onset: _____

_____

_____

_____

_____

_____

MY DETAILED HEALTH PROFILE

Respond to the questions to add valuable information to your health inventory.

How old were you when you had your first period?

_____

_____

Have you gone through menopause? If so, at what age?

_____

_____

Do you have diabetes, prediabetes, or insulin resistance? If yes, indicate which one and, if known, the results of your most recent HbA1c test. _____

_____

_____

Blood pressure: Note your systolic (the top number) and diastolic (bottom number) numbers from your latest blood pressure reading: Systolic _____ Diastolic _____

Have you been diagnosed with high blood pressure?

_____

Do you or an immediate family member have high cholesterol or triglyceride levels? _____

_____

Do you smoke or vape? _____

Do you live in a household where others smoke? _____

Do you engage in regular physical activity for thirty minutes or more every day? _____

Are you currently experiencing stress? If yes, please indicate the cause. _____

_____

_____

_____

Do you sleep for at least seven hours every night? _____

_____

Have you or a first-degree member of your family been diagnosed with an autoimmune disease (lupus, rheumatoid arthritis, etc.)? _____

_____

_____

_____

Have you been diagnosed with any of the following pregnancy-related complications: gestational diabetes, gestational hypertension, preeclampsia, or eclampsia? _____

_____

_____

_____

Have you been diagnosed with other gynecologic conditions, such as polycystic ovary syndrome or early menopause? _____

_____

_____

_____

Have you been diagnosed and treated for breast cancer? What type of treatment? _____

_____

QUESTIONS FOR YOUR HEALTH PROVIDER

Use this space to jot down any questions you'd like to ask your health provider. Take your completed health inventory with you to ensure that you are receiving the best and most informed care.

At my next appointment, I would like to ask my health provider about the following: _____

_____

_____

_____

_____

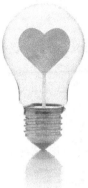

Chapter Four

KNOW YOUR SCORE: YOUR PERSONAL RISK FACTOR ASSESSMENT

All of the recent studies confirm that heart disease can be prevented or controlled with the following:

- Awareness, knowledge, and ability to put into action those lifestyle changes that prevent or control the risk factors that lead to heart disease or that eliminate the issues that already caused a heart attack

- Partnering with your doctor to develop a personalized plan for risk-factor identification and modification

- Adherence to all medically prescribed recommendations, including medications taken regularly, as prescribed

The following questions will help you assess your personal risk of heart disease. Check the box next to "Yes" or "No" after each question.

MY PERSONAL RISK FACTOR ASSESSMENT

These are risk factors for heart disease you cannot control (nonmodifiable risks).

Race and Gender

I am Black or Latina or South Asian.

☐ Yes
☐ No

Age

I am fifty-five years or older.

☐ Yes
☐ No

Menstrual History

I am postmenopausal or had surgically induced menopause.

☐ Yes
☐ No

I went through menopause before the age of forty.

☐ Yes
☐ No

Family History / Genetics

I have/had a male relative with heart disease before age fifty-five.

☐ Yes
☐ No

I have/had a female relative with heart disease before age sixty-five.

☐ Yes
☐ No

Next are the modifiable risks—the risk factors that you can control:

Pregnancy Issues

During one or more pregnancies, I had gestational diabetes (elevated blood sugar), preeclampsia, eclampsia, a preterm delivery, or elevated blood pressure.

☐ Yes
☐ No

Blood Pressure

I am being treated for high blood pressure or my BP was 140/90 or higher on two or more occasions (or 135/85 if diabetic).

☐ Yes
☐ No

Diabetes

I have diabetes, or I have been told that my blood sugar is too high.

☐ Yes
☐ No

Cholesterol

My cholesterol level is _____.

My HDL (high-density lipoprotein) is less than 50 mg/dl.

☐ Yes

☐ No

My LDL (low-density lipoprotein) is greater than 100 mg/dl.

☐ Yes

☐ No

My triglycerides are greater than 150 mg/dl.

☐ Yes

☐ No

BMI

I have a BMI (body mass index) of twenty-five or more.

☐ Yes

☐ No

Waist Circumference

My waist measures more than thirty-five inches.

☐ Yes

☐ No

Cigarette Smoking

I smoke cigarettes or vape.

☐ Yes

☐ No

I live or work with people who smoke cigarettes in my presence.

☐ Yes
☐ No

Physical Activity

I get less than thirty minutes of physical activity on most days of the week.

☐ Yes
☐ No

Autoimmune Diseases

I have been diagnosed with rheumatoid arthritis, lupus, or another autoimmune condition.

☐ Yes
☐ No

Stress/Lifestyle

I feel stressed much of the time.

☐ Yes
☐ No

I am always on the go, with little or no time for myself.

☐ Yes
☐ No

I can get overwhelmed with a sense of foreboding (doom and gloom).

☐ Yes
☐ No

Sleep

I routinely get less than seven hours of sleep a night.

☐ Yes

☐ No

Totals: Yes _____   No _____

Understanding Your Score

Look at your total score. Every yes in the category of modifiable risk factors indicates an area where you have an opportunity to make changes to get your health on track. We recommend that you take this list to your doctor, along with your Personal Health Inventory, so that he or she can help you customize a program that focuses on specific areas in which you need help. Your doctor can also fill in the blanks if you were unable to answer any of the questions, such as those asking for cholesterol or blood pressure numbers. Going forward, make sure you know these important numbers.

If you did mark yes to any of these questions but are thinking, "I feel fine. Why do I need to make any changes?" remember that heart disease begins silently and can remain hidden for years; you may not know the impact of your risk factors until it's too late. Our goal is to help make sure that does not happen to you. As we've told you throughout this book, it is never too late to begin your journey to heart health.

REMEMBER THAT HEART DISEASE BEGINS SILENTLY AND CAN REMAIN HIDDEN FOR YEARS; YOU MAY NOT KNOW THE IMPACT OF YOUR RISK FACTORS UNTIL IT'S TOO LATE.

Risk Factors for Heart Disease in Women: A Recap

As a reminder, keep in mind these key risk factors that may apply to you:

- Family history of premature heart disease in a first-degree relative—parent or sibling—before age fifty-five in a male relative or at age sixty-five in a female relative.

- Race or ethnicity (higher for Black, Latina, and South Asian women)

- Age (higher for women over the age of fifty-five)

- Prediabetes: HbA1c of greater than 5.7 percent

- Diabetes: HbA1c of greater than 6.5 percent

- Hypertension: BP higher than 120/80 mm Hg

- Abnormal cholesterol/triglyceride levels

- Obesity, especially where the bulk of weight is in the waist/ midsection ("apple shape")

- Cigarette smoking or frequent exposure to secondhand smoke

- Physical inactivity (sedentary lifestyle)

- Early onset (before age forty) of menopause from any cause

- Stress

- Lack of adequate sleep

- Systemic autoimmune disease (e.g., lupus, rheumatoid arthritis)

- A history of pregnancy-induced diabetes, hypertension, pre-eclampsia, or eclampsia

Congratulations—you've begun to gather the information you'll need to become smarter about your heart and to begin to make progress toward a healthier you! Now that you have begun to identify your potential risk factors and have completed your personal health inventory, it's time to learn more about the clues and cues your own body is providing.

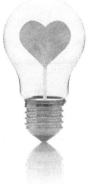

Chapter Five

PAY ATTENTION TO THE CLUES AND CUES: YOUR BODY TELLS A STORY

Claudia

Remember Claudia, the forty-eight-year-old Puerto Rican woman we introduced in chapter 1? As you will recall, Claudia is a high-level banker with a stressful career and a busy home life. As luck would have it, her symptoms of exhaustion, heart palpitations, shortness of breath, and changes in her usually calm demeanor coincided with her annual checkup with her primary care physician.

Claudia described her diminished energy and other symptoms to her doctor. The doctor conducted a thorough examination, which included a complete battery of blood tests. Her doctor noted that this was the second time that Claudia's blood pressure had been elevated in the office and performed a treadmill exercise stress test to see if elevated blood pressure with exercise was the cause of her symptoms.

After eight minutes on the treadmill, the test was stopped due to Claudia's fatigue and very elevated blood pressure. Her doctor placed her on medications to control her blood pressure and recommended that she come back in three months for a follow-up visit.

Claudia resumed her busy schedule, took her blood pressure medication, and gradually returned to exercising on the treadmill for thirty minutes a day five times a week. She continued to have diminished energy, and she noted a slight change in her usually sound sleep pattern. She was having trouble falling asleep and on a few occasions awakened suddenly, feeling anxious for no apparent reason. She attributed her sleep disturbance to anxiety about her upcoming trip to Hong Kong, where she was going to close a huge financial deal.

It was two months after her stress test that we met Claudia in the emergency room. On that day, she had returned from her four-day trip to Hong Kong and had gone directly from the airport to her office. However, right away she began to experience overwhelming fatigue and severe shortness of breath. In addition, she was sweaty and had mild chest discomfort. She told her coworkers she was sure it was just jet lag, but they didn't agree and called 911.

Tests in the emergency room indicated an abnormal electrocardiogram, a sign that she might be on the verge of having a heart attack. A coronary angiogram (X-ray of the coronary arteries) revealed plaque in the heart's large coronary arteries, with a clot creating a significant blockage in a branch of one of the main arteries. Claudia underwent an emergency procedure to place a stent (a small, tube-shaped device) in the artery to keep it open and increase blood flow to her heart, thereby avoiding the possibility of an imminent heart attack. As she lay in the recovery room, Claudia recalled that both her mother and her older brother had had a stent implanted, for similar reasons.

It is possible that Claudia's stressful schedule, the fourteen-hour flight with little sleep, and dehydration precipitated the clot formation and led to the symptoms that brought her to the emergency room. But going to the emergency room and having the stent procedure performed less than three hours from the onset of her first symptoms probably saved her life! That blocked vessel could very well have caused a heart attack.

The sequence of events leading up to her emergency stent procedure made Claudia reflect on the important clues her body was providing that she had either missed completely or passed off as unimportant. She now understood that her body was signaling that something was seriously wrong. She realized that her mother's and brother's history of heart disease, her own elevated blood pressure, and the constant stress caused by family life and work all placed her at risk for heart disease. Once she began experiencing a noticeable decrease in her ability to exercise, a feeling of fatigue while walking, and episodes of shortness of breath for no apparent reason, she should have recognized that those were all clues and cues that she had heart disease—clues and cues that she ignored.

Trust Your Intuition!

Heart disease warning signs can be subtle. Women often ignore what they think are minor aches and pains, but you need to know that if something doesn't feel quite right, it probably isn't. Trust your intuition—make a doctor's appointment and get yourself checked out. If you suffer from one or more of the symptoms listed later in this chapter, it could be

> **YOU NEED TO KNOW THAT IF SOMETHING DOESN'T FEEL QUITE RIGHT, IT PROBABLY ISN'T.**

an early warning sign of cardiac disease. Call your doctor right away. Do not hesitate, because your life could depend on it.

Work with Your Doctor to Establish a Personal Baseline

There are many early warning signs of heart disease that often go unnoticed, and the best way to determine the significance of these symptoms is to visit your doctor. If you are having symptoms, and these symptoms are due to heart disease, you can be treated, and if they are not, then your doctor can use the visit to establish a baseline to assess any future symptoms. If you are not having symptoms, your annual well-woman visit will provide your doctor with an opportunity to screen you for any evidence of heart disease or heart disease risks (see Week 4 of the Six S.T.E.P.S. in Six Weeks Program). Being aware of how your body feels and functions when it is in a healthy state allows you to recognize anything you experience that is out of the ordinary. When you are tuned in to your normal everyday aches, pains, sleeping patterns, and activity thresholds and are aware of how you normally react to work and family stress, you and your doctor will be more aware of and better able to judge the seriousness of any symptoms you may be experiencing, and you will be in a much better position to know when to consult your health provider.

Developing an ongoing partnership with your healthcare provider and knowing your baseline are of critical importance for all women but especially for those of you who already have any of the risk factors for heart disease. If this describes you, be especially vigilant about monitoring your health and reporting any and all changes, no matter now minor you think they are, to your healthcare provider.

The Signs and Symptoms of Ischemic Heart Disease or Heart Attack

Recognizing the signs and symptoms of ischemic heart disease or heart attack may be challenging when it comes to women. Even today, when we know so much more about women's heart attacks, many doctors tend to focus on the most common symptom (in both men and women): chest pain or discomfort. But this is problematic for women, since many of them do not exhibit this symptom, and therefore a heart attack can go undiagnosed.

That is why you need to advocate for yourself and help your doctor diagnose your heart attack. It could save your life. Remember, too, that you can experience *any* of the common symptoms listed below, days, weeks, or months before a heart attack actually occurs. Some of these symptoms may seem so benign that you want to brush them off. Don't. Seemingly benign symptoms like shortness of breath, a passing pain in the chest, heartburn, nausea, and vomiting, and back or jaw pain may not seem like emergencies, but if they tend to recur, call your doctor and get checked out. Always err on the side of safety.

The Most Common Symptoms for Women

While many men and women experience chest pain or chest pressure that radiates to the left arm as the main sign of a heart attack or of ischemic heart disease, the following symptoms are far more common in women than in men and can lead to an underappreciation by both women and their clinicians of the likelihood of heart disease. As you look at this list, it's important to remember that every woman is different; some may experience only one of the following signs, some may experience more than one sign, and 40 percent may experience no chest pain at all.

- **Uncomfortable pressure, fullness, squeezing sensation or pain** anywhere in the chest or back. These symptoms may last only a few minutes or longer; they may persist or occur sporadically. None of these symptoms is normal in a healthy woman.
- **Mild or intense pain that begins in the chest and spreads to the shoulders, neck, jaw, or arms** (left or right side). This type of pain is more common in women and can come on suddenly (and can even wake you up), or it can come and go before getting more intense.
- **Unexplained dizziness, lightheadedness, or fainting.** These symptoms may or may not be accompanied by palpitations.
- **Shortness of breath or difficulty breathing with or without discomfort in the chest.** This feeling can be experienced alone or may be combined with nausea or lightheadedness.
- **Clammy sweating.** This is the type of sweating that comes with feeling anxious or stressed out; it feels different from sweating when you are experiencing a hot flash, are in a warm place, or are exercising. Breaking out in a nervous/cold sweat is a symptom very common in women who are having a heart attack.
- **Stomach pain, abdominal pressure, or nausea** that may feel like common indigestion, the flu, or a stomach ulcer but can also feel like a weight sitting on your stomach.

- **Back pain** that may mimic muscle pain related to overexertion.
- **A feeling of weakness or fatigue or the inability to perform even simple tasks or activities.** The onset of any of these symptoms may or may not be sudden and without any obvious cause. They are sometimes combined with vague feelings of lack of mental sharpness and that something is "just not right."

When to Call 911

If you are experiencing these symptoms and think they may represent a heart attack, call 911! Time is a crucial factor when dealing with a heart attack. The sooner you get help, the better your chances of a full recovery. Call 911 immediately if you experience any of these symptoms—no matter how subtle—and say out loud to yourself or anyone around you, "I think I am having a heart attack." Trust your gut feeling. Never second-guess yourself. Do not wait for the pain or strange feeling to pass.

Under no circumstances should you attempt to drive yourself or allow anyone else to drive you to the hospital. You need to be in an ambulance! The sooner you get medical help, the better your chances of survival. If you are having a heart attack, your treatment will start the moment the ambulance arrives. Your life may depend on it.

Then, before the ambulance arrives, if you know you can safely take aspirin, *chew* one full-strength aspirin tablet (or three low-dose tablets), with or without water. If you are alone, be sure that the door is unlocked. Sit down and rest until the ambulance arrives.

Evaluate Your Lifestyle to Make Meaningful Changes

Be honest with yourself. As you read earlier, Claudia believed that she was living a heart-smart life. She was careful to maintain an exercise regimen that included aerobic activity and strength training. She kept an eye on the scale to make sure her weight stayed within five pounds of her prepregnancy weight. She took good care of her appearance, and everyone told her how great she looked. Heart disease was not on her radar!

But what Claudia failed to realize was that she needed to be more honest with herself and to delve more deeply into her family history and her daily routine to see what she needed to change. Fortunately for Claudia, before she left the hospital, the medical team assisted her in this process. They helped her recognize that despite the fact that she exercised regularly and maintained a healthy weight, she had other risk factors that contributed to her visit to the emergency room.

These habits included eating fatty "comfort" foods such as steak, cheese, cookies and chips when traveling. The constant stress of dealing with the competing demands of her job and family—long hours of travel, soccer games, homework, and housework—had taken its toll. As if this wasn't enough, Claudia put pressure on herself to always bring her A game and to be as close to perfection as possible in everything she tackled. All of these things were major contributors to her heart disease.

With the help of her medical team, Claudia was able to develop a plan like the one you are about to learn, one that focuses on the important changes needed to prevent a heart attack.

When it comes to our approach to food, exercise, sleep, and stress management, we can all make small changes in our daily routines and habits, and these small changes can yield meaningful results. As you will see when you read on, the Six S.T.E.P.S. in Six Weeks Program we have designed will jump-start your journey to heart-smart living. Like Claudia, you'll be surprised at how simple it can be.

Let's get started!

PART TWO

SIX S.T.E.P.S. IN SIX WEEKS TO A HEALTHIER HEART

"I have been impressed with the urgency of doing. Knowing is not enough; we must apply. Being willing is not enough; we must do."
—LEONARDO DA VINCI

The goals of our Six S.T.E.P.S. in Six Weeks Program are to give you the tools to better understand your personal health status and to encourage you to partner with your physician and take an active role in your own health and well-being. We want you to feel empowered to make the small changes that can lessen your chances of ever developing heart disease.

Know that whoever you are, we are cheering for you as you begin this program! Choosing to live a healthier life is an important choice and a powerful choice.

As you get started, and throughout the program, you may need additional tips, more resources, or even the encouragement of a community of women just like you who are choosing to live a heart-healthy life. You'll find helpful resources at the end of this book and also on our website. Get connected and share your story!

It is important that your health is always your top priority, so we have designed a program that is easy to follow and easy to live with to help you accomplish that goal. Each week you'll have the opportunity to begin to practice new ways of thinking, and experiment with different choices, in a specific area of your life. Remember, this is *your* program and your opportunity to choose to live a healthier life. This isn't a diet or a short-term fix. You're making choices and taking the slow, deliberate steps toward a life that is healthy, energetic, and balanced.

Let's begin by taking a big-picture look at the program. Each week has a specific focus. The last week, Week 6, shows you how to put it all together and take permanent S.T.E.P.S. to your healthier life.

WEEK 1, S: Select and stock the kitchen with healthy food choices.

WEEK 2, T: Take control of your activity and choose to move every day.

WEEK 3, E: Eat for a healthier heart.

WEEK 4, P: Partner with your doctor, family, and friends.

WEEK 5, S: Sleep more, stress less, and savor life.

WEEK 6, Put it all together: Permanent S.T.E.P.S. to a Healthier Heart.

That's the heart of the program, six steps in six weeks. Our hope is that you'll find encouragement on these pages—and plenty of knowledge. This is the information you'll need to make smarter choices when you shop for food, when you move through your day, when you plan meals, when you take care of your body—even when you sleep. These are the smarter choices that will ultimately equip you to be *heart smarter.*

This is your program, and this is your book. Make notes on the pages and track your progress. If you find a message that encourages or inspires you, write it in the margin or at the top of the page! Tear out the shopping lists, highlight the new foods that you've tried and loved. We want this book to tell your story as you live a heart-healthier life.

Are you ready to get started? We can't wait to share these steps with you! Just a few final tips before you begin the Six S.T.E.P.S. in Six Weeks Program:

Tip #1: Choose a Teammate

This program is easy to follow, but because all journeys are easier and more enjoyable with the company of a friend or family member, we strongly encourage you to ask someone close to you to help on this journey. Choose someone who can offer you moral support and encouragement, share in your successes, and provide a friendly ear if you are finding it difficult to stay on course, someone who can laugh with you and compliment you when you make progress, someone who can be counted on to share and celebrate your triumphs and prop you up when you slip. In short, someone who will always be there for you.

The best partner won't just be your cheerleader—they'll be a teammate. If you and your teammate are both working toward these same heart-health goals, you can share suggestions and solutions. Two people going through the same experiences together can have a very powerful and positive effect on each other.

Tip #2: Keep a Notebook/Journal/Smartphone Log

You're starting a new adventure—you'll want to keep a record. The powerful sensation of making positive change. The energy you experience. The recipes you try that are delicious—and yes, the epic fails. The way you feel on day one and the way you feel at the end of six weeks.

A journal is the optimal tool to track your progress as you begin this health journey, and it will be helpful for years to come. Purchase a journal that you like and find easy to use, because it's going to be your lifelong companion. Treat yourself to a beautiful hardcover journal or, if you prefer, pick up an inexpensive spiral notebook at the dollar store. Look for one with dividers to help you get organized. You can also set up your journal on your smartphone, computer, or tablet. You'll want to track your progress consistently, so choose the platform that is easy for you to use, one that you'll reach for every day. This simple journal will become the most important asset on your road to a healthier heart in ways you can't yet imagine. Charting your progress will help you stay motivated. In the moment, you may not see progress or change, but your journal will show just how far you've come. Keeping a record allows you to remember this entire journey—and document your accomplishments and challenges.

> **TWO PEOPLE GOING THROUGH THE SAME EXPERIENCES TOGETHER CAN HAVE A VERY POWERFUL AND POSITIVE EFFECT ON EACH OTHER.**

What should you include in your journal? First, customize it to make it truly yours. Add the words and images that will encourage you and inspire you. You'll want to include your Personal Health Inventory in an easy-to-find section, most likely the beginning of your journal. We discussed the importance of this earlier in the book—remember, taking the time to compile this record is a key step in taking responsibility for your health and will ensure that you have the data you need in one central place.

If you haven't compiled your Personal Health Inventory, now is the time! Get your journal, and get started with the following:

- Family medical history, including a general look at your family's health (e.g., mother had cancer at age fifty-seven, brother has had hypertension since age forty-three, etc.)

- Your medical history (pregnancies, surgeries, procedures and hospitalizations, as well as chronic conditions)

- Allergies (including details about the type of reaction you may have had)

- Current medications and vitamins/supplements (including dosage and frequency)

- Previous regimens of medication, vitamins/supplements, and all other over-the-counter products (including any reactions or side effects)

- If relevant, your age when you gave birth and your age when you experienced menopause

- Race and ethnicity

- Smoking history

- Any physical activity habits (how many times per week and for how long—fifteen minutes, thirty minutes, an hour)

- Stress in your life

- Autoimmune diseases

- Pregnancy-related risk factors (gestational diabetes, gestational hypertension, preeclampsia, eclampsia)

- Recent medical tests (including HbA1c, blood pressure, cholesterol levels)

- Weight

- BMI

- Waist circumference

It's a good idea to set aside a section of your journal for listing the questions you want to ask your healthcare professional during your office visit or on the phone. Be sure to leave enough space to note the answers and any special instructions. It's very common to feel nervous during an appointment with a doctor. Write down your questions before the appointment, and keep your journal handy so that you can make a note of the answers when the appointment has ended.

Your Personal Health Inventory will be a valuable resource for your doctor and healthcare team, so bring it with you to every appointment. Even if you are seeing several doctors within the same healthcare system, your medical records might not be shared between physicians. You are responsible for keeping your medical team up to date, and the most efficient and effective way to do this is to provide them with the information from your Personal Health Inventory.

And speaking of your healthcare professional team, before you start the program, as you should before starting any type of health program, *get checked out by a* clinician. Explain that you are starting a new program. When you go for this first visit, take your journal along. Be sure you've filled in your list of personal risk factors and as much of your Personal Health Inventory as possible. Armed with this information, you will be well on your way to becoming an active partner with your doctor. We'll talk more about this valuable partnership in Week 4.

You've identified a teammate. You've consulted a doctor or nurse practitioner. You've set up your journal and are ready to note your progress, identify setbacks and successes, and track questions or concerns you need to raise with your healthcare professionals. One last tip:

Tip #3: It's OK to Look Back

Your journal will be a great way to track your progress, so don't be afraid to look back. Be sure to set time aside to read over what you've written. It will encourage you, remind you of things you may have forgotten, and help you stay on track with your health. You may choose to share your journal with your buddy for his or her input, but this is a record especially written by you, for you.

You've made a powerful and courageous choice—the choice to live a healthier life. Now, let's get started!

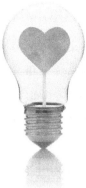

Week 1

S: SELECT AND STOCK YOUR KITCHEN WITH HEALTHY FOOD CHOICES

To create a heart-healthy environment at home, and to be able to set a healthy table, you'll need to make decisions about choosing healthy foods. It's simple: if you want to eat foods that are good for you and good for your heart, you want to surround yourself with great options—and get rid of any unhealthy foods that will make it harder to make good choices.

What you have in your house right now may not live up to heart-smart standards, so during this first week, we'll go through your kitchen, see what needs to be eliminated, and then offer suggestions on what you can buy to replace those less healthy items. Think of it as spring cleaning for your kitchen—we'll get rid of the clutter that no longer fits your new lifestyle to make room for some wonderful new choices.

Clean Out Your Refrigerator

The key to heart-healthy living is knowing which foods are good for you to eat and which are not. Take stock of the contents of your refrigerator. Go ahead—open that refrigerator door and take a careful look. What do you see? Do you find whole milk, butter or margarine, ketchup, creamy salad dressings, fruit juice, sodas, cream cheese, pizza, processed cheese slices, hot dogs, salami and other deli meats, bacon, teriyaki sauce, pickles, or jellies and jams? Now, check the freezer. There you may find more high-fat, sugar- and sodium-laden leftovers, along with ice cream, ice pops, frozen pizza, fish sticks, chicken nuggets, convenience meals, frozen pancakes, and more.

The foods that we just listed are the foods you are going to get rid of, because all are high in fat, sugar, and/or sodium. Check the labels. Learn which foods in your refrigerator and freezer are "ultraprocessed" foods and should be purged. Ultraprocessed foods are foods that contain ingredients that are not typically used when cooking from scratch, such as artificial sweeteners, colors, or flavors or other additives. If the label contains a long list of ingredients that you can't pronounce—ingredients that you don't recognize as actual food items—it's likely that you're holding something that's been ultraprocessed. Some examples of ultraprocessed foods are soft drinks, many sugar-sweetened cereals, chips, chicken or fish nuggets, instant soups, and boxed rice mixes or mac and cheese, just to name a few. These foods are loaded with chemical additives and are often high in sugars, saturated fats, and sodium, all of which contribute to heart disease. The bottom line is that these foods are generally high in calories and low in nutrients and have no place in a heart-healthy kitchen.

In most cases, there are healthier alternatives to all of these foods that will keep you satisfied and that you will enjoy so much that you won't miss the unhealthy foods you used to eat. But right now, your goal is to get rid of all the harmful foods listed above. Any food that is high in refined carbohydrates (meaning they are made from enriched white flour or wheat flour), unhealthy fats, or sugar should be purged from your kitchen. From now on, the goal is to focus on buying and eating flavorful, healthy foods.

Purge the Pantry

Now, move on to the cupboards, the pantry, wherever you store food. It's time for another long, careful look, just like you did in the refrigerator and freezer. Push aside the cans and boxes that are in the front to see what you've accumulated over the years (yes, years). If you're like the rest of us, you may find a few packages of food that have stayed there so long, they should be paying rent.

It's time to get rid of those cans and boxes and packages that are simply taking up space. The best way to do this is to pull everything out and separate the items that are unhealthy and anything that has expired. Now, you're ready to purge! Toss out any expired food right away. Next, identify and toss all of the unexpired foods that are no longer on your heart-healthy menu. This includes things like salted pretzels, chips of any kind (potato, taco, corn, veggie, etc.), packaged cookies and refined crackers, cakes, pies, cake or cookie mixes, bouillon, full-fat baking mixes, chocolates and candies, boxed rice mixes, canned soups, macaroni and cheese, baked beans, syrup, etc. You get the idea. All of the ultraprocessed foods in your pantry should be purged. Packages of baked goods, snacks, and desserts are generally ultraprocessed, but check the label's first three ingredients. If some form of added sugar or fat is listed in the top three, it no longer belongs in your house.

START YOUR PURGE HERE

To jump-start your pantry purge, here are some unhealthy foods that you'll want to immediately usher out of your kitchen. If you find any of these unwanted guests in your refrigerator, freezer, or cabinets, say a quick farewell and toss them out:

- Margarine/shortening/lard/butter
- Whole milk / cream / cream cheese / sour cream
- Soda / diet soda / fruit punch / sweetened beverage mixes
- Candy and chocolates
- Chips and salted pretzels
- Frozen pizzas / french fries / frozen entrées / frozen vegetables with added sauces
- White bread / rolls / muffins / croissants / bagels
- Hot dogs / deli meats / Spam / bacon
- Boxed macaroni and cheese and rice mixes
- Packaged cookies, cakes, and pastries

Create Your Healthy Food Makeover

Now that you have purged your refrigerator, freezer, and pantry of the unhealthy foods, it's time to restock your home with healthy foods. Set up a shopping list using your journal or phone. You'll want plenty of delicious options, so stock your refrigerator and pantry with as many of these as your budget permits.

YOUR ESSENTIAL SHOPPING LIST

These are the items that should be in your shopping cart during your next trip to the grocery store:

- ☐ Plenty of fresh fruits: Apples, kiwi, pomegranates, berries, melons, etc.
- ☐ Vegetables: Cauliflower, kale, spinach, broccoli, radish, cucumber, tomatoes, brussels sprouts, mushrooms, bok choy, sweet potatoes, etc. (plain frozen veggies are a great choice too!)
- ☐ Olive and extra-virgin olive oil, avocado, walnut, and flax oils
- ☐ Salmon and other cold water fatty fish, canned salmon, sardines, or tuna (low-sodium varieties)
- ☐ Whole-grain and sprouted grain breads, pasta, crackers, flour, and cereals (read those labels!)
- ☐ High-fiber foods like beans, dried peas, lentils, and chickpeas ("pulse" foods)
- ☐ Brown rice, wild rice, whole wheat couscous, quinoa, farro, bulgur, and other whole grains
- ☐ Raw, unsalted nuts (almonds, cashews, hazelnuts, pecans, walnuts, etc.)
- ☐ Unsalted seeds (sunflower, hemp, pumpkin), chia seeds, and ground flax
- ☐ Low-fat or fat-free dairy products (or unsweetened, nondairy alternatives)
- ☐ All-natural peanut and nut butters (look for 100 percent nuts and no extra sugar)
- ☐ Eggs and/or pure liquid egg whites
- ☐ Skinless chicken breast and extra-lean ground chicken and turkey

Your Heart-Smart Shopping List

In the box, we've provided a list of essentials as a quick reference, but on the pages that follow we'll spend a little time building your shopping list in more detail to help you understand the many delicious options available—and why they matter. At the end of the book, we'll share a week's worth of menus using many of these ingredients to help inspire you.

You may want to invest in organic options or prefer a plant-based, vegetarian or vegan diet. You can use these building blocks to create a customized meal plan that works for you. You'll experience more success if you make sure that you have plenty of options—a rainbow of fruits and vegetables, a variety of lean sources of protein, and healthy solutions when you're hungry and need a quick meal or snack.

So read through these ideas, circle the items that you want to try, and build your own shopping list. The list that follows is only the beginning. More and more healthy options appear on the grocery shelves every day, so read those labels. You'll be surprised at the available variety of food that is good for you.

DAIRY AND EGGS

From now on, choose to eat low-fat (1 percent) or fat-free (0 percent) milk or unsweetened dairy alternatives such as soy milk, milk made from nuts (almond, cashew, etc.), or hemp or oat milk, to name a few. If you are buying cow's milk, stay away from half-and-half, "whole" or full-fat milk, and reduced-fat (2 percent) varieties. These are just too high in fat. That also goes for cheese and yogurt. It might take a few tries to find the brands you and your family prefers, and they may cost a bit more, but it's worth the investment. Once you discover healthy new foods that you enjoy, you will never feel deprived. Please do not give up! Changing your eating habits is an adjustment and will take a little getting used to. It might be just that you are unaccustomed to less sugar, salt, and fat in your diet. So be patient while your taste buds adjust.

If you are lactose intolerant or simply prefer one of the plant-based "milks," you are lucky to be living in a time where you can choose a milk made from soy, almond, cashew, oats, hemp, or rice, among others. Some of these taste like the milk we all know, and some are flavored (avoid the ones with added sugar), adding a nice touch to cereal or a cup of coffee. Again, try different brands until you find the ones you like best, and look for brands without unnecessary additives like carrageenan, an added emulsifier or thickener used to improve texture. Although carrageenan is on the FDA's GRAS (Generally Regarded as Safe) list, there is some concern that it may cause gastrointestinal discomfort.

While you're in the dairy section, don't forget eggs. The latest research says that if your LDL cholesterol is within healthy limits, you do not have to eliminate the yolks as long as you eat eggs in moderation. Also, remember to prepare your eggs without added saturated fats and avoid eating them with high-fat foods such as bacon or toast with butter. Eggs also make a great foundation for added veggies, so try making an omelet or scramble with your favorite vegetables!

We find that it's always good to have a container of liquid egg whites on hand (and an extra container in the freezer), as they are versatile. You can scramble them or make an omelet or frittata, and you can use them in baking and cooking.

MEAT, POULTRY, AND FISH

Meat, poultry, and fish are high in protein and other important nutrients and are an integral part of a healthy eating plan, so leave room in your freezer to stock these items. We'll talk a bit more about portion sizes for these foods in Week 3, but meat, poultry, and fish can still be part of your life if you simply commit to a few smart choices.

When it comes to meat, choose the leaner cuts, and look for "round" and "loin" cuts like top or bottom round, sirloin, filet mignon, pork tenderloin, or boneless center-cut pork chops. Remember to always trim off the visible fat before cooking. Ground beef should be lean 92/8 (which means 92 percent lean / 8 percent fat); or even better, buy extra-lean 96/4 (96 percent lean / 4 percent fat). Stay away from the fatty meats, which include pork bacon, ribs, pork shoulder chops and roasts, marbled steaks, chuck roasts, and ground chuck. Lamb is also a good option when you choose lean cuts from the leg and loin. Avoid cuts from the rib and shoulder blade, which are higher in fat. A three-ounce cooked lean cut of meat contains, on average, less than 10 grams of fat, less than 4.5 grams of saturated fat, and less than 95 milligrams of cholesterol. An even better option is to purchase grass-fed, grass-finished beef, which is leaner than traditional grain-fed beef. Grass-fed means the cattle consumes grass, not grain products. This results not only in a more nutrient-rich product; it can also have five times more omega-3s than conventional beef. Still look out for those leaner ratios for grass-fed ground beef as well.

Fish should definitely be a part of your diet; we recommend eating it at least twice a week. All unprocessed fish is good, but focus on eating mostly fatty fish like salmon, mackerel, lake trout, and herring because they are higher in omega-3 fatty acids, as opposed to fish like catfish or crawfish. Canned fish is also a healthy choice, so stock up on mackerel, sardines, salmon, and tuna (packed in water, and low-sodium varieties). Remember that, with fish, the preparation matters. You don't want to turn a healthy food into an unhealthy one! Avoid frying fish, fish sticks, or prebreaded varieties, which are often high in added sodium and added fats. Instead, try steaming, grilling, baking, and broiling your fish. Experiment with different cooking techniques, and discover how they change the way the fish tastes. Identify a few methods that you love—fish cooks quickly, so it's a great choice for a quick and healthy meal.

Most types of shellfish—clams, oysters, mussels, scallops, lobster, crab, and shrimp—are a good choice for lean protein since they are low in saturated fat. While shellfish, particularly shrimp, contain higher amounts of cholesterol, new guidelines suggest that dietary cholesterol has little effect on blood cholesterol levels, so moderate consumption of any type of shellfish should not be a problem (just be sure to avoid dunking it in butter). Once again, pay attention to your preparation: shellfish is no longer heart-healthy if it's prepared with ingredients high in saturated fats (think shrimp or lobster in cream or butter sauce, or fried fish and chips). Avoid frying shellfish and cook it in a healthier way, with little added fat and without rich cream and butter sauces.

> REMEMBER THAT, WITH FISH, THE PREPARATION MATTERS. YOU DON'T WANT TO TURN A HEALTHY FOOD INTO AN UNHEALTHY ONE!

While fish is a heart-healthy food, there are some concerns that we want to address. Some species are overfished, and some are high in heavy metals and toxins. While we encourage you to consume fish regularly, it would be wise to select fish that are sustainably sourced and are not high in mercury and other toxins. What does this mean? Start by staying away from swordfish, shark, king mackerel, gulf tilefish, marlin, and orange roughy, which are all high in mercury, and limit canned tuna to no more than two eight-ounce cans per week. Certain farmed fish, such as farmed salmon, contain polychlorinated biphenyls, which may contribute to cancer risk. The Monterey Bay Aquarium's website is a great resource to learn more about the fish you're purchasing and whether or not it's sustainably sourced: www. seafoodwatch.org.

We've spent a lot of time talking about fish and meat. Poultry is another good choice for a heart-healthy diet. Chicken breast and turkey breast cutlets are excellent sources of protein with very little fat. If you're choosing ground chicken or turkey, read the label and make sure that you buy the brand with the lowest fat content. Use ground chicken breast and extra-lean ground turkey breast, which is 99 percent fat free. Lean ground turkey is also a better alternative to ground beef, but be aware that this product can often be a combination of white meat, dark meat, and skin, making the fat content a bit higher at 93 percent lean / 7 percent fat. When using whole chicken parts, be sure to remove the skin before eating. The leanest choice would be skinless chicken breast.

Sausage? Yes—provided that you choose sausage made from healthy meats. You'll find many varieties of sausage made from either turkey or chicken. They're lower in fat than the pork varieties—and they taste delicious.

FRUITS AND VEGETABLES

When you go to the grocery store, your first stop should be the fruit and vegetable aisle. Fruits and vegetables should always be the first item on your shopping list, and should be front and center in every meal you eat. Fruits and vegetables are chock full of vitamins, minerals, and fiber and have proved beneficial in preventing or treating disease. You'll want a variety of colors because the different colors are offering you different vitamins and minerals. Fill your shopping cart or basket with dark leafy greens, orange and purple carrots, red peppers, brightly colored apples … you get the idea! Fresh and plain frozen varieties are ideal. While it's our least favorite option, when buying canned fruit (which is typically lower in fiber), make sure it's packed in natural juices or water, not syrup.

Keep your refrigerator full of raw vegetables and fruit for healthy snacking and add fruit to every meal for a naturally sweet dessert. There are no bad choices when it comes to this food group, so this is a great place to experiment and try new things. Remember, too, that some vegetables, like the leafy green varieties (kale, spinach, Swiss chard, broccoli rabe, etc.), are also high in iron and taste great.

Organic produce is wonderful, but it can be more expensive. A healthier diet is one that's lower in pesticides and chemicals, so one alternative is look for local farmers markets or produce stands, where fruit and vegetables have been grown locally and don't need the chemicals and preservatives required when food is shipped longer distances.

Another option is to splurge on organic items when it matters most—on the fruits and vegetables more likely to contain higher quantities of chemical residues and pesticides. When following a budget, buy conventional produce for fruits with thick peels, like bananas or oranges. The Environmental Working Group (ewg.org) has published a "dirty dozen" list—this can be a helpful resource if you want to minimize your exposure to pesticides. When your budget permits you to splurge on organic produce, start here:

- Strawberries

- Spinach

- Kale, collard, and mustard greens

- Nectarines

- Apples

- Grapes

- Cherries

- Peaches

- Pears

- Bell and hot peppers

- Celery

- Tomatoes

WHOLE GRAINS, BEANS, AND LENTILS

Whole grains, beans, and lentils should all be part of your staple diet. Quinoa, spelt, flax, chia, barley, and farro are all ancient grains that are making a comeback as part of the thoroughly modern diet.

And now, a word about pasta: When it comes to pasta, steer clear of refined white carbs and try the newer whole-grain versions, which have gotten a lot tastier over the past few years. Look for pastas that are made from 100 percent whole grain. Or check out the new pastas made from chickpeas, quinoa, brown rice, or red lentils. In some grocery stores, you'll find these in the gluten-free or organic aisles. Don't be afraid to experiment, and remember to stick to recommended serving sizes, because pasta is a type of carb you can easily overeat. Substituting zucchini noodles or spaghetti squash is another great way to sneak more veggies and fiber into your diet.

When buying bread, cereal, pastas, and flours, always choose high-fiber, whole-grain varieties. There's even white, whole-grain bread that has a mild flavor and soft texture—a good choice for picky kids. When it comes to rice, stay away from white and choose brown or wild rice. When choosing a nutritious, high-fiber cereal, you cannot beat that old standby, oatmeal, especially the steel-cut variety. If you buy the instant oatmeal, make sure it is the plain variety with no added sugar. You can always add your own fruit, such as bananas, apples, peaches, pears, or berries (fresh, dried, or frozen) and/or a sprinkle of cinnamon to make it tastier without adding sugar. For an even better fiber boost, top with some almonds or walnuts too!

WHOLE GRAINS: CHECK THESE OUT

You may be wondering exactly what are all of these whole grains we keep referring to. If you are only thinking whole wheat, you're thinking too small! There are many whole-grain options that you can try. On your next shopping trip, look for these new grains—and try a few:

- ☐ Amaranth
- ☐ Barley
- ☐ Buckwheat (soba noodles)
- ☐ Brown or wild rice
- ☐ Chia
- ☐ Corn
- ☐ Freekeh
- ☐ Flax
- ☐ Millet
- ☐ Oats
- ☐ Sorghum
- ☐ Spelt
- ☐ Teff

- ☐ Quinoa
- ☐ Triticale
- ☐ Whole-grain rye
- ☐ Whole wheat (spelt, emmer, farro, einkorn, kamut, wheatberries, bulgur)
- ☐ Whole wheat flour and whole wheat pastry flour

Don't be fooled by vegetable chips, which are often mostly dyed potatoes, or crackers "made with" whole grains. No matter their name or their claim, fried chips (potato, taco, corn, and their cousins) and crackers are not part of a healthy diet. Take a careful look at the label, and you'll see that they are often much too high in fat and salt.

Beans and Lentils

Beans and lentils (including the canned variety) are an excellent component of a healthy diet. They are nutrient dense (meaning they have high amounts of nutrients per calorie), are high in protein, carbohydrates, fiber, vitamins and minerals, and are low in fat. If you are eating canned beans, remember to rinse them well to remove as much sodium as possible.

CONDIMENTS/FLAVORINGS

Some condiments are high in sugar, fat, and sodium. Ketchup, for example, can be very high in sugar and sodium, but there are now low-sugar or no-added-sodium options available. Excellent condiment choices are mustard, vinegars, salsa, and hot sauce, which tend to be fat-free and can be used to dress up a variety of foods.

Not all salad dressings and barbecue sauces are created equal; some can be high in sugar, fat, and sodium. Mayonnaise should be used sparingly; choose one of the healthier varieties made with canola, olive, or avocado oil. For an even healthier option, substitute low-fat Greek yogurt in recipes. For salad dressings, read the labels and choose the lighter varieties. Pay attention to the serving sizes; a healthy choice may be as simple as using a measuring spoon to control your portion size. Better yet, make your own with a cold-pressed extra-virgin olive oil and vinegar.

Fruit jellies, jams, and preserves also fall into this category; all traditionally made varieties are made up of almost half sugar. For this reason, we suggest limiting your consumption and buying the fruit-only varieties. They taste exactly the same and are much healthier. Even better, smash your own fresh fruit to make your own natural spread!

SALT

To add flavor to foods, don't rely on salt—in fact, we suggest that you take the salt shaker off the table! We get enough sodium in our diet naturally from food and from those hidden sources of sodium in packaged or prepared foods. To bump up flavor, try a salt substitute, cook with garlic, use lemon juice and lemon zest, and don't be afraid to experiment with spices and herbs. Try one of the many packaged spice and herb combinations (but make sure to read the label and only buy one with no added salt), or make your own.

CAN-DO CONDIMENTS

On your next shopping trip, add these condiments to your list:

☐ Mustard

☐ Ketchup (low sugar and/or low salt)

☐ Vinegars (balsamic, apple cider, red wine, etc.)

- ☐ Salsa
- ☐ Hot sauce (including sriracha)
- ☐ Dried spices without additives (such as cinnamon, thyme, basil, parsley, red pepper, cumin)
- ☐ Tahini
- ☐ Citrus fruits (e.g., lemon, lime, or orange zest or juice)

BEVERAGES

When it comes to nonalcoholic beverages, the choices are pretty simple.

Anything containing sugar is out. This includes any full-sugar sodas, fruit nectars, and fruit juices. You should be eating fruit, not drinking it. If you like your beverages flavored, that's not a problem. You'll find many fruit-flavored and no- or low-calorie sparkling waters on the supermarket shelves. Or make your own soft drink by splashing a bit of fruit juice into a glass of plain seltzer, squeezing in a wedge of lemon, lime, or orange or infusing other fresh fruit or mint. Cucumber water is particularly refreshing!

We do not recommend drinking diet soda. If you can't give up diet sodas and beverages completely, which is ideal, choose to identify soda as the special treat it should be. Reduce your intake and treat yourself only once in a while, because many recent studies actually link diet soda consumption to weight gain as well as high blood sugar.

Coffee and tea are back on the recommended food list, and caffeine isn't an issue unless it keeps you up at night. Flavored and herbal teas are always a good choice, as is green tea with its own health benefits.

DRINK ME

These beverages will always be your best choices—they provide us with fluids, without added sugar or calories:

- Water (add flavor with a spritz of citrus, or infuse with fruit)
- Sparkling water or seltzer
- Unsweetened coffee or tea

A note about your morning cup of joe. If you're accustomed to having your coffee or tea light and sweet, we recommend you gradually reduce the amount of sugar you add. The end goal is no added sugar at all. It may take your taste buds time to adjust, so be patient and consistent. Be sure to use real milk (or your preferred nondairy alternative) rather than coffee creamer. Most are made from oil, sugar, and preservatives. We encourage you to read those ingredients. You will be very surprised.

When it comes to alcoholic beverages, red wine has recently been given the distinction of being a heart-healthy addition to the diet. Red wine contains polyphenols that may reduce the risk of stroke and heart disease by protecting the lining of the blood vessels in your heart. However, it is important to note that this means "moderate" wine consumption, which for women is one five-ounce serving per day. It is not recommended that you start drinking wine if you don't already do so, and if you do drink, don't increase the amount you drink. If you abstain from alcohol, you can get heart-healthy benefits from other sources of polyphenols, such as green tea, red or black grapes, and even a small square of dark chocolate of 70 percent cacao content or higher.

With respect to other types of alcohol, such as beer and hard liquor, avoid drinking to excess. Too much alcohol has been associated with raising triglycerides and contributing to weight gain and obesity. And most cocktails are prepared with a lot of sugar. If you choose to drink, avoid sugary cocktails and instead choose one serving of the following: wine (five ounces), beer (twelve ounces), or hard liquor (one ounce).

SWEETENERS

It is best to limit the amount of sugar in your diet, particularly refined white sugar, but regardless of the source, sugar is sugar. *We recommend that you steer clear of all artificial sweeteners.* If you are cooking or baking, there are many all-natural sugar substitutes to try, some of which even provide nutritional benefits. Experiment with some of your favorite recipes by replacing part of the sugar with dates, molasses, agave, honey, coconut sugar, or maple syrup (pure, not artificially flavored). Keep in mind, albeit natural, these are still a source of added sugar in the diet and should be used sparingly.

OILS, BUTTER, AND BUTTERY SPREADS

Monounsaturated oils such as olive, canola, peanut, and safflower are all heart-healthy. Newer on the supermarket shelf is avocado oil, a heart-healthy oil for cooking as it has a high smoke point. A fruity olive oil can be pricey, but it is healthy and delicious in a salad dressing or when used sparingly as a substitute for butter. Make sure to select extra-virgin olive oil that has been cold-pressed to get the most polyphenols and superior taste. To cut down on fat and calories, use a spray mister to coat the pan when cooking, or use it to spray over salad greens. Other healthy polyunsaturated fats to include on your shopping list are walnut oil and flax oil, both great-tasting options for dressings and marinades!

We've never met a person who didn't like butter, but butter consumption should be limited. A little dab is OK here and there, but don't overdo it, and try to use whipped butter versus stick. A pat of butter has 2.2 grams of saturated fat, and you should aim to use less than 15 grams total of saturated fat per day. You may think margarine is a better choice, but stick margarines contain partially hydrogenated oils, and some tub margarines have just as much saturated fat as butter. Although margarine does not contain cholesterol, it does contain fat and calories. If you must use margarine, read the label and choose the one with the lowest saturated fat that is trans fat–free. There are plenty of buttery spreads on the supermarket shelf made from heart-healthy oils from which to choose.

Heart-Smart Pantry Staples

Are you ready to get started on stocking your pantry with heart-healthy food? The following is our recommended list, the items you'll want to add to your shopping list. When you open your refrigerator, your freezer, or your pantry, these are the foods you should find. This list is by no means complete, but it will guide you in choosing the healthy foods to have on hand so that you can create a range of well-balanced meals or treat yourself to a healthy snack:

- Whole wheat flour or almond flour

- Cornmeal

- Cereals (oatmeal and any other cereals with five or more grams of fiber, three grams or less of fat, and no more than five grams of sugar per serving)

- Whole-grain or sprouted-grain breads/crackers

- Brown or wild rice

- Whole-grain pasta (whole wheat, brown rice, quinoa or bean/lentil-based pastas)

- Whole-grain side dishes (quinoa, spelt, flax, millet, farro, barley, etc.)

- Spaghetti sauce (low sodium, low sugar)

- Canned tomatoes (whole, diced, or pureed)

- Coffee and tea

- Soups and broths (low sodium)

- Canned fish (salmon, herring, tuna, sardines, and mackerel) packed in water, olive oil, or tomato sauce

- Oils for cooking and salad dressings (avocado, olive, canola, extra-virgin olive oil, walnut, flax)

- Beans and lentils (dried or canned)

- Fruits and vegetables (fresh or frozen)

- Ketchup (low sugar or low salt)

- Mayonnaise (made from olive, avocado or canola oil)

- Mustard / salsa / hot sauce (to dress up meat, fish, potatoes, eggs)

- Salad dressings (low sugar / light)

- Vinegar (for homemade dressings)

- Healthy snacks (whole-grain crackers, unsalted pretzels, graham crackers, plain popcorn)

- Almonds, cashews, pecans, walnuts, hazelnuts (raw, unsalted, or plain dry roasted)

- Nut butters with no added sugar or salt (almond, peanut, cashew, or sunflower)

Take a picture of the list with your phone and keep it handy every time you go to the store. Use it as your guide as you try new foods. Make a note of what you love (and what you don't!).

Before this week ends, we have a few more tips to share:

Shop the walls of the grocery store. Produce, meats, fish, dairy, bread, and deli products are stocked along the outside walls of the supermarket. When you shop the perimeter of the store, you won't be tempted by the unhealthy foods that you are trying to avoid, so hug those walls! If you must pass through the bakery department, pick up some tasty whole-grain bread.

Always read the labels. Many packaged foods have surprising amounts of sodium, sugar, and/or fat. For example, spaghetti sauce, bread, cereal, yogurt, and marinades can have added sugar. If you see any of the following listed on a food label, know that the body processes all of these as sugar, because that is what they are: maltose, fructose, high-fructose corn syrup, dextrose, lactose, sucrose, molasses, cane sugar, corn sweetener, raw sugar, white granulated sugar, brown sugar, sugar, powdered sugar, invert sugar, fruit juice concentrate, applesauce, syrup, honey, malt syrup, maple syrup, nectars.

Make a shopping list. Make a list, buy only what's on it, and don't browse! Doing this will save you money, calories, and time. It's also a good idea to list your purchases in categories and in the order in which the foods are arranged in your particular market. Most stores have an app or a digital shopping list option on their websites. Or use the list we've provided in this book!

Eat before you go shopping. Have you noticed that it's difficult to stick to your shopping list if you're hungry? Try to do your food shopping *after* you have eaten. Shopping when hungry will result in too many impulse items, often high in fat and sugar.

Stock up. If you can, shop for the coming month. The idea here is to develop your own system of planning meals and then shopping for the ingredients. When you stock up, you'll always have groceries on hand and will be less likely to run out for fast food. Now that you've cleaned out the pantry and know what foods you need to eat, get the family involved and plan ahead.

Demonstrate healthy eating habits. Getting healthy is a family affair, and you are all going to be eating the same food. (Granted, the kids may still get an occasional sugary snack, but limit these to teach them healthy eating habits.)

Get family members involved. Chances are your family members have a favorite type of food that they cook well, so you can enhance the cooking and shopping experience by assigning a day of the week to cook for the family to each member of your household who wants to cook. Your role will be to point out some healthy options. For those who are too young to cook, ask for their suggestions and get them involved by shopping and maybe even helping with the preparation— even if it's only setting the table. These types of activities that are centered around meals encourage family members to become active participants in creating, cooking, and serving heart-healthy foods they like to eat, and you get the bonus of having the family sit down together for a meal.

If you live alone, partner with a couple of friends or relatives and cook for one another. In this case, the choice of meal is up to the cook. Or each of you can make a meal and package and freeze it for each member of your group. Set aside a day to exchange these pre-portioned meals so that each of you will have multiple heart-healthy meals in your freezer. If you're partnering with a teammate as part of this journey to heart health, this is a great activity you can share to support and encourage each other.

Create a meal-planner notebook. We have found that using a meal-planning app or a notebook that has dividers or tabs you can designate for breakfast, lunch, dinner, desserts, and snacks will help you keep track of your favorite recipes as well as the ingredients needed to prepare them. Doing this offers the added advantage of providing space to write comments on the recipe, such as "Maria really liked this" or "Easy to make." At the end of this book, you'll find a week of sample menus to get you started.

Congratulations! You have begun a brand-new set of habits and behaviors this week! Take a moment to celebrate this milestone. Make a note in your journal of anything about the week that has surprised you. Reflect on how you are feeling, and allow yourself to feel proud of the positive changes and healthier choices you've made this week.

Now on to Week 2, where you'll have the opportunity to begin to practice a new habit that will keep your heart healthy: adding exercise to your daily routine.

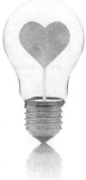

Week 2

T: TAKE CONTROL OF YOUR ACTIVITY AND CHOOSE TO MOVE EVERY DAY

Now that you have stocked your pantry with heart-healthy foods, it is time to incorporate a daily activity routine into your heart-healthy lifestyle. In this chapter, we will focus on three types of activity:

- **Walking:** The health benefits of aerobic activity and how to meet your goals

- **Strength and flexibility training:** The importance of strong and flexible muscles

- **Moving:** The significant health benefits of choosing to just "move" more in your everyday activities

Remember, you're beginning to make new choices and practice new behaviors. You're learning how to live a healthier life! Your goal should be to move—and then to move a bit more. If you choose to join a gym or devise a formal exercise program to follow at home, that's great! But the goal is to ensure that aerobic activity, strength and flexibility training, and simply moving more throughout the day are all part of your life.

Research has shown that the simple act of walking is "the closest thing we have to a wonder drug," according to Dr. Thomas Frieden, former director for the Centers for Disease Control and Prevention.[12] In order to maximize the health benefits of walking, your goal should be to incorporate a good walk into your daily routine. Do you need to drive to work—or can you walk? Instead of driving your kids to the bus stop, walk with them. Start small, and add a few steps every day.

As you choose to move more, get creative and think of ways to add other types of aerobic activity to your daily life. Pull out that old bicycle (the one you rode around the neighborhood when you were a teenager, or the stationary one that now sits idle in your bedroom closet) and go for a spin. The same goes for that treadmill gathering dust. Find an exercise class—in person or online—and try it out. The purpose of this chapter is to give you a framework and some suggestions to get you on the road to incorporating these three elements into your daily life: walking, flexibility and strength training, and just plain moving.

Focusing on your heart health means embracing a more active lifestyle and, in the process, discovering the incredible benefits of activity. The great thing about being more active is that you will experience the benefits almost immediately. When you are active, your body is moving in a higher gear, your heart is beating faster, and oxygen-rich blood is being pumped through your body and nourishing your organs and your brain. You think more clearly, sleep better,

---

12   "Vital Signs: Walking among Adults—United States, 2005 and 2010," CDC, August 10, 2012, https://www.cdc.gov/mmwr/preview/mmwrhtml/mm6131a4.htm.

and have more energy. The more energy you expend, the more you will have. Your joints will lubricate and your muscles will stretch—and you'll feel better physically, emotionally, and mentally. Being more active will energize your life.

But first things first! As mentioned, be sure you get a checkup from your clinician before you begin any type of exercise program—including a walking regimen. Your doctor or nurse practitioner will let you know if you have any limitations, and if

> **FOCUSING ON YOUR HEART HEALTH MEANS EMBRACING A MORE ACTIVE LIFESTYLE AND, IN THE PROCESS, DISCOVERING THE INCREDIBLE BENEFITS OF ACTIVITY.**

you do, pay attention to them and don't try to push past them. As you build stamina, your threshold will increase. Be patient.

Walking

THE BENEFITS OF WALKING

What if we told you that we had a great new exercise that was easy to do, required no expensive equipment, and could be done anytime and anywhere? All of us learn to walk as toddlers, so by now you have decades of experience with this "wonder drug." We agree that it is the perfect way to get your daily dose of activity.

Numerous studies confirm the health benefits of walking. One important example is the landmark Harvard Nurses' Health Study, in which the health behaviors of over two hundred thousand women were studied for more than thirty years. This study showed that walking at a moderate pace for an average of thirty minutes each day can lower the risk of heart disease, stroke, and diabetes by 30 to 40 percent and the risk of breast cancer by 20 to 30 percent.

WALK ON!

Here's even more encouragement to get you to lace up those walking shoes and head for the door:

- Walking helps to lower blood pressure.

- Walking improves balance and bone strength (thereby reducing the likelihood of falls and fractures).

- Walking counteracts the effects of weight-promoting genes.

- Walking improves your sleep.

- Walking boosts your mood.

- Walking sharpens your thinking.

- Best of all, walking is gentle on your knees and the rest of your body.

Consider this: an eight-year study of more than seventy thousand women found that brisk walking and vigorous exercise substantially reduced the incidence of heart attacks.[13] What's more, even light to moderate activity—a minimum of one hour a week—was associated with lower rates of heart disease.

No matter how busy you are, you can find an hour a week for a walk. But increase that number to 30 minutes per day and your risk of premature death will be significantly lower than if you didn't exercise at all.

---

13   F. B. Hu et al., "Walking Compared with Vigorous Physical Activity and Risk of Type 2 Diabetes in Women: A Prospective Study," *JAMA* 15 (October 20, 1999): 1433–39.

SETTING GOALS FOR YOUR WALKING PROGRAM

Your goal should be to work up to walking thirty minutes each day at a pace that is "moderate" or "purposeful." Think of the pace at which you would walk to a meeting if you were running a few minutes late, a pace at which you could carry on a conversation but with a bit of difficulty. That's what we mean by a moderate pace. You will get your heart rate up and will experience the benefits of aerobic activity.

What is aerobic activity? Aerobic activity is sometimes referred to as "cardio," and it includes any brisk activity that stimulates and strengthens the heart and lungs, thereby improving the body's use of oxygen.

HOW TO BEGIN A WALKING PROGRAM

The Physical Activity Guidelines from the US Department of Health and Human Services recommend that adults get 150 minutes of moderate aerobic exercise each week, and we want you to target that amount as your ultimate goal. However, for those of you who have not been exercising on a regular basis, we recommend starting slowly—and checking with your doctor before you do. Begin with three to five minutes of moderate or "purposeful" walking each day. This should translate into three to three and a half miles per hour in order to get your heart rate to where it should be. Be sure to warm up and cool down for two to three minutes.

After you have completed week one of your walking program, increase the purposeful walking component by five minutes, and continue to do that each week until you reach twenty minutes of purposeful walking each day (with an additional five-minute warm-up and a five-minute cooldown).

For many of us, it's easier to use an app on our phones to count steps and set daily goals to move more. If that's you, we recommend starting with three thousand steps and gradually working your way up to ten thousand steps each day.

Need help getting started? Here are a few thirty-minute solutions, ideas you can use to get in your thirty minutes of walking every day:

- Take a walk after dinner or lunch.

- Take public transportation one stop before or beyond your usual stop.

- Walk before work or walk to work, if that's possible (ditto the walk home).

- Enlist a family member or neighbor to join you for a walk.

- Walk your dog or volunteer to walk a neighbor's dog.

- Take the long route when walking anywhere (including the mall).

- Join the morning walking group at your local mall (call the mall to get the time).

- Head to the local elementary or high school and walk around the track.

Set a goal for this week of trying as many of these as you can. Check them off when you do!

It's important to remember that significant benefits are to be had even if you are not able to meet these goals. Any additional activity is a *step* in the right direction! Just to recap, here are the benefits of walking each day:

- Lowered blood pressure

- Reduced risk of heart disease and certain types of cancer

- Increased joint and muscle strength and flexibility

- Increased bone strength

- Increased energy level

- Improved sleep

WHAT TO WEAR: DRESS FOR WALKING COMFORT AND SAFETY

Dress for the temperature, but be sure you have good socks and shoes and a bra that supports you well. Everything you wear has to fit well, be comfortable, and not bind or chafe. You don't have to invest in expensive workout clothing. Walmart, Target, and thrift stores all sell workout clothes. Just don't skimp when it comes to walking shoes. Good shoes keep you in balance by supporting your ankles, knees, and back, and they also make your feet feel good, and that's important. You need the benefits of a walking program to maximize your health, so buy the best pair of shoes you can afford!

SAFETY TIPS

A few tips to keep you safe as you begin your walking program:

- When walking during hot weather, dress in lightweight and light-colored clothing.

- Don't forget to wear sunscreen and sunglasses.

- Never leave home without a cell phone.

- If walking after dark, wear reflective clothing and/or a clip-on light or carry a flashlight.

- Make sure you always tell someone where and when

you will be walking and when you expect to be back. So many people forget this step!

- Enlist the company of a friend or family member to make walking more enjoyable and safer. This is a great activity you and your teammate can share!

- Adhere to the rules of the road by using sidewalks and crosswalks and obeying traffic signals.

- When on rural or suburban roads, always walk facing oncoming traffic (unless you are walking up a hill or around a blind bend) so you can see what is coming and have time to get out of the way, if necessary.

- Always walk in familiar places where you know you will be safe.

Learn to Monitor Your Heart Rate

As we mentioned earlier, it is important to get approval from your doctor or nurse practitioner before beginning any exercise routine. Once you have the go-ahead, you will need to learn how to monitor your heart rate to ensure that you are getting the most out of your workout. If you are new to exercise, you may not be accustomed to the feeling of your heart working at increased capacity. You may feel that you are getting lots of exercise as you go up and down stairs at work or walk around the mall, but unless you properly monitor your heart rate, you won't know for sure. Depending on a number of physical factors including weight, overall health, muscle condition, and blood pressure, you could be working your heart too hard, or not hard enough, without even knowing it.

KNOW HOW HARD YOUR HEART IS WORKING

You can't tell how hard your heart is working by how much you sweat. Even while working out at the same intensity, some women are drenched while others are barely damp.

That's why it's important to monitor your heart. Heart monitoring calculates the intensity of your workout by actually counting the number of heartbeats per minute (BPM). Exercise makes the heart beat faster, making it work harder to deliver the increased blood and oxygen demanded by the muscles during a workout.

To exercise safely, you should stay in a "zone" between 50 and 85 percent of your *maximum target heart rate,* which is defined as the absolute highest rate a heart should beat during exercise at a specific age. As a general rule, your maximum heart rate is approximately 220 minus your age.

Unless you are a professional athlete in training, your heart should never beat as fast as the maximum rate. Because heart rate is related to age and because the heart slows slightly as we age, our target zone beats per minute will decrease as we age. Below is a chart created by the American Heart Association to help you determine your target heart rate zone, counting BPM:

Age	Target Heart Rate Zone	Maximum Heart Rate
20	100–170 BPM	200 BPM
30	95–162 BPM	190 BPM
35	93–157 BPM	185 BPM
40	90–153 BPM	180 BPM
45	88–149 BPM	175 BPM
50	85–145 BPM	170 BPM
55	83–140 BPM	165 BPM
60	80–136 BPM	160 BPM
65	78–132 BPM	155 BPM
70	75–128 BPM	150 BPM

Reference: American Heart Association, https://www.heart.org/en/healthy-living/fitness/fitness-basics/target-heart-rates.

Knowing your range helps you determine how hard you should be exercising and when you are overdoing it—or not pushing yourself enough. When first starting your exercise regimen, aim for the low end of the zone, and as you build stamina and add more intense workouts, aim for the higher end of the zone. You may wish to check with your clinicians to see if you have any personal limitations before determining the heart rate you should aim for.

HOW TO MEASURE BPM

Every beat of your pulse is a beat of your heart. The easiest way to accurately count the number of times your heart is beating per minute is to check your pulse. Gently place your forefinger and middle finger on the inside of your opposite wrist. Hold your finger there for fifteen seconds, counting the beats. Then take that number, multiply it by four, and you will have your BPM.

You should take your pulse periodically as you exercise. Practice taking your pulse manually. There are also apps you can download that can measure BPM using your smartphone or tablet.

Strength and Flexibility Training

As we now know, aerobic activity is essential for good heart health. However, in order to ensure that you embark on an exercise program designed to improve your overall health, it is important to add some resistance, or strength, training as well as flexibility exercises to your weekly routine. This will help you build muscle mass, strengthen your bones, and improve your metabolism. Strength training enhances the benefits of aerobic exercise. It is important to include twenty to thirty minutes of strength and flexibility training in your exercise routine at least two times per week.

To begin your strength and flexibility program, you will need a few basics.

EQUIPMENT

Exercise/yoga mat. A soft surface will make exercising more comfortable. You can purchase a mat at a discount or sporting goods store.

Weights. Many strength-training exercises can be done with no equipment at all! Using only your own body weight, you can do planks, push-ups, wall push-ups, squats, abdominal crunches, and more. But if you would also like to use weights for strength training, we recommend two dumbbells (two to five pounds each). If you don't have dumbbells, don't worry—you can make your own! Take two empty one-liter water or soda bottles and fill them with water or sand. Better yet, use two plastic half-gallon milk bottles (with convenient handles, which make them easier to hold on to and manipulate). To make them lighter, reduce the amount of water or sand; you can add it back as you gain strength.

If you do decide you want to use dumbbells, by all means get them. You needn't purchase new ones. They can often be found in a thrift or used sporting equipment store. Initially, five pounds each should be your limit. They may not seem heavy enough, but once you start lifting them multiple times, you will see that they are!

Resistance bands. These are stretchable bands that provide resistance when stretched. You can find them in any sporting goods store.

You'll find suggestions of a simple strength-training workout that can be done almost anywhere, with no equipment other than a chair and your body weight, later in this book.

FLEXIBILITY EXERCISES

Stretching is an important part of any exercise routine. It is recommended that you perform flexibility exercises for all of your major muscle groups: upper body (shoulders, chest, arms) and lower body (glutes, adductors, hamstrings, quadriceps, and calves). Later in this book, you'll find some suggestions for flexibility exercises for each of these major muscle groups.

MOVING—TEN MINUTES AT A TIME

Even if you are a seasoned exercise buff, you can probably find more opportunities to move throughout the day. The goal is to take every opportunity to keep your body *moving*, rather than remaining sitting or standing still. Prolonged sitting can be damaging to your health, even if you already exercise on a regular basis. Here are some

> TAKE EVERY OPPORTUNITY TO KEEP YOUR BODY *MOVING*, RATHER THAN REMAINING SITTING OR STANDING STILL.

suggestions that we hope will get you thinking of even more ways to add movement to your day:

- Park your car farther away from your office, the bank, the store, etc.

- Pace the room while you're on the phone or watching TV.

- Stand up and march in place each time a commercial comes on.

- Take the stairs instead of the elevator or get off a floor or two earlier (or more, if you are able) and walk the rest of the way.

- Walk up the escalator or along the moving sidewalk—don't stand still.

- Use the bathroom one floor up or down at work and take the stairs.

- Get up from your desk at least once every hour to stretch your legs for a minute or more.

- Do a few minutes of yard work (pull a few weeds, rake a bit, sweep the sidewalk).

REMEMBER TO HYDRATE

Making sure you drink enough water is always important, but remember to drink even more when you exercise. The body can become dehydrated for a number of reasons. Sweating is the major reason during exercise, but you can also get dehydrated when it's cold outside and you are not sweating. Exercise causes the body to dehydrate no matter what the temperature.

So make it a point to drink an eight-ounce glass of water about ten minutes before you walk or exercise and another glass or two when you finish, no matter what the season or temperature. In addition, you should get into the habit of always having a bottle of water handy to sip throughout the day, no matter what the temperature and no matter where you are, to help you stay hydrated.

SET ASIDE A SPECIFIC TIME AND PLACE TO EXERCISE

Make an appointment to exercise—and make sure that you keep it! Write it in your calendar, or set a reminder on your phone or computer. Choose any time of the day that works best for you and when you won't feel pressed for time. For indoor exercising, find a place where you have the space to lift your weights and keep your "exercise stuff" together. The point is to make this as easy and fuss-free as possible. You need to be able to just walk to your space and start exercising. Maybe there is space in front of your TV—if so, consider doing your workout while watching your favorite show. Do whatever it takes to make this as enjoyable as you can.

There are many videos and books to help you map out a personalized exercise routine. There is not one "right" video or routine; try as many as you want to keep yourself interested and to make it fun.

Log Your Progress

Keeping track of your exercise progress will prove invaluable to you on your road to heart health. Not only will you be able to look back and see how far you've come, but it will also make it easier to set realistic goals for yourself as you continue with your exercise program. Record keeping will encourage you to keep going and to take pride in your accomplishments. There are many different ways to log your progress, so choose the one that works best for you.

Here are a few examples you can use to track your exercise progress. Test a few different options to find the one that you can use consistently and easily—that way, you know that you'll keep better records of what you've accomplished!

IN YOUR JOURNAL

Use your trusty journal. Add a section to keep track of your strength training progress, and simply note the number of reps you do for each exercise, gradually increasing the number of reps (until you reach ten to twelve) or the amount of weight (if you are using dumbbells or ankle/wrist weights).

Use a pedometer or other fitness tracker to count your steps, and note them in your journal. The advantage of using a pedometer (or phone app, which we'll discuss later) is that it will count all of your steps during the day, not only the steps you take when walking or exercising. Up and down those stairs, back and forth to the kitchen and bathroom, to and from your car—all those steps add up. Aim for 3,000 steps a day to start and increase gradually until you get to 10,000 (about five miles) per day. (Figure that there are roughly between 2,200 and 2,300 steps per mile.) You can also download a walking journal or workout template from the internet. Search for "free walking log," "free walking journal," or "exercise log," and you'll be directed to many sites where you can choose the type of log or journal format you prefer, print out the blank template, and insert it into your journal.

GO DIGITAL

Because your goal this week is to choose to move more, you'll want to be able to easily and quickly measure your progress. Keeping track of your walking progress is effortless if you wear an activity tracker or smart watch or use a phone app that electronically maintains a log for you. All that is required is an initial setup of the application or device. If you want to buy an activity tracker but aren't exactly sure if one is right for you, read on and also check them out in person at any sporting goods, electronic, or department store.

The biggest boon to fitness in general, and walking in particular, is the tracker. Perhaps you've seen these brightly colored rubber bracelets with flashing lights on people's wrists. A basic tracker (which generally sells for about $100) is preset to a goal of ten thousand steps, or five miles per day. But that number can be adjusted higher or lower, depending on where you are in your walking goals. They can be a great motivator and may be worth the investment. In addition to counting steps, these basic trackers can monitor hours slept and keep track of calories and ounces of water consumed. More sophisticated models alert for email or text messages, tell time, monitor heart rate, and count number of stairs climbed or laps swum. The Apple Watch is a more expensive option—with more features—but a basic pedometer works perfectly well if your goal is just to count steps.

When you opt to wear an exercise tracker, you will have an easy way to keep an accurate record not only of how many steps you've taken but also of the duration and intensity of your movement. This way, you will know just how much of your walking is moderate or purposeful as opposed to simply strolling.

These devices take the guesswork out of keeping track of your movement, but they cannot do the work for you. What they can do, however, is motivate you into action and keep you going. They're a great way to maintain a log of your daily activity and monitor your progress. Some can even be set to reward you with "prizes" when goals are met or exceeded.

Like to be social? Some trackers and phone apps allow you to incorporate social networking elements so that you and your friends, colleagues, or family members can register on their website as a "group" that will post progress of each member. If you aren't comfortable with having people you know see your progress, you can be measured against strangers who have registered but wish to remain anonymous as well. This friendly competition can prove to be a real motivator.

If you already own a smartphone and don't want to go to the expense or keep track of another electronic device in your life, then download one of the many free apps. Many have monitoring capabilities similar to those of the fitness trackers, and some are more sophisticated than others. Don't be afraid to try out different ones until you find the one that best suits your needs.

If you're turned off by the appearance of the solid-colored rubbery wristband, there is good news! You can find beautifully colored and decorated wristbands for many varieties of trackers, most modestly priced at just a couple of dollars. Some are more sophisticated in their design and actually look like bracelets, which makes them wearable with even the trendiest outfits. Fashion plus fitness: a great combination!

Once you get hooked on the positive feedback you get from your device, it will be hard to stop wearing it. Twenty-four hours a day, this little device is capable of motivating you and keeping track of how much you've slept, how much ground you've covered, how many calories you've eaten and burned, how many pounds you've lost, how far away you are from your target weight ... they even reward you when you reach daily or long-term goals. If you have had trouble motivating yourself to exercise, a fitness tracker may provide the push you need to get going. If you're the competitive type, it will keep upping the ante and raising your goals. No matter how you look at it, these devices make striving toward a healthier and more active life easier.

But the bottom line is that whatever device you opt for—whether an app, a fitness tracker, a pedometer, or simply notes in your journal—it's all up to you to start moving. You can do it!

Other Types of Exercises

Although our focus here is on walking, strength training, and flexibility exercises, there are countless other activities that can provide an excellent workout. Jogging, swimming, cycling, rowing, tennis, skating, skiing, and basketball are just a few aerobic activities that will contribute to your heart health. Learn to monitor your pulse while you engage in these activities to ensure that you are within your target heart rate zone.

Movement Matters

The most important advice for you to take away from this section is that *any movement or activity that you add to your daily routine is beneficial to your heart health*. If you have not previously included exercise as part of your daily regimen, start slowly. Gradually work up to the goal of thirty minutes of moderate aerobic activity each day, with additional twice-a-week strength and flexibility exercises. Every day, set a goal to take one more step, add a bit more weight, or walk for a few more minutes. Keep track of your progress and note what works for you and what doesn't. Most importantly, enjoy yourself.

KEEPING TRACK

Use this worksheet to keep track of your progress—and show you how much you have to celebrate! We've given you space to update this information as often as you want.

My daily step count: _____

_____

My goal this week is to walk for this many minutes: _____

_____

I'll add ten more minutes of movement to my day by this date: _____

_____

This week, I am choosing to practice this strength exercise:

_____

_____

This week, I am choosing to practice this flexibility exercise:

_____

_____

At the end of this week, take time to reflect in your journal on how far you've come since you started the program. Make a note of all of the changes you've made. Celebrate your progress. Every step is a step toward a heart-healthier life.

Now, on to Week 3 and learning how to eat heart smart.

Week 3

E: EAT FOR A HEALTHIER HEART

In Week 1, you stocked your pantry, refrigerator, and freezer with healthy items. This week, we'll spend some time focusing on how to use those wonderful ingredients to eat a delicious variety of heart-healthy meals.

Week 3 is presented in two parts because the subject of eating is of such major importance when it comes to maintaining heart health. We have separated the basic guidelines for setting a healthy table from the rules for healthy eating, both at home and when dining out.

Part One: Find a Healthy Balance

You have achieved so much already! Your kitchen is stocked with healthy foods, and exercise is becoming part of your daily life. So let's now turn to the subject we all love—eating. In the first section, we focus on the basic rules for healthy eating and how to do that without denying yourself your favorite or comfort foods. You will see how easy it is to eat in moderation and prepare familiar or traditional foods in healthy ways. You'll also learn which foods are best for keeping your heart healthy and your body satisfied.

EATING TO LIVE, NOT LIVING TO EAT = HEALTHY EATING

We all need to eat in order to stay alive, but when we live to eat—well, that's what gets us in trouble. However, eating to live also means knowing how to choose tasty foods that will be calorie friendly and good for our blood pressure, arteries, and any health conditions we may have, such as diabetes, heart issues, or obesity.

This sounds simple, but if you already have health problems, you may have a complicated relationship with food that interferes with making healthy choices. Our health depends on the foods we choose to put in our bodies. What we eat can either harm our health or keep us healthy. All the medicine in the world can't overcome the effects of an unhealthy diet. But once you know the basics for making healthy food choices, you'll be on the road to heart health.

WHY EATING IS EMOTIONALLY COMPLICATED

Many of us come from families that equate food with success and happiness. We all had a mother, grandmother, or aunt who wasn't happy unless we ate everything on our plate, whether we were hungry or not. Perhaps they told you stories of the starving children who would have gobbled up the food we left on our plates. Or maybe you learned to "medicate" with food. When you were unhappy, food was your reward—perhaps an ice cream cone, a slice of cake or pie, or a candy bar made you feel better. If you felt lonely, maybe eating a dish of spaghetti, macaroni and cheese, or a pepperoni pizza did the trick. We all have our traditional favorites, and we tend to eat them in large portions and not always cooked in a healthy way. Complicated relationships with food are common, but now it's time to begin to try different behaviors as we begin to understand the health consequences attached to not paying more attention to what we put in our mouths.

Our goal is not to analyze all of the psychological forces at work when it comes to your eating habits. But we can help you prepare, serve, and eat familiar and satisfying foods in healthier ways and in healthier portion sizes, which will improve and maintain your heart health.

A WORD ABOUT DIETS

It seems that every other day we hear of a new diet that is getting press. Remember, diets are not necessarily heart-healthy because they are popular, nor do they tend to promote long-term sustained weight loss. Any diet that restricts whole food groups or one that cannot be sustained long-term is not something we recommend.

That's why we encourage you to think about forming new healthy eating habits and creating heart-healthy meal plans, rather than talking about diets or deprivation. But there are two "diets" (eating styles) that may help you jump-start healthier eating that we'll highlight here: the DASH diet and the Mediterranean diet. These are the most highly recommended and sustainable for heart health.

DASH Diet

As you practice new eating habits and experiment with incorporating healthier food choices into your diet, you may it find it helpful to explore the DASH diet.

DASH stands for "Dietary Approaches to Stop Hypertension," and as its name suggests, it's an eating plan designed to reduce your blood pressure by encouraging you to eat foods that are low in saturated fat, total fat, and cholesterol and to increase your consumption of fruits, vegetables, and low-fat dairy foods. A DASH diet includes plenty of whole grains, poultry, fish, and nuts while limiting your fats, red meats, sweets, and sugared beverages. In short, it's a lot like the tips we're recommending in this book!

In a study published by the *Journal of the American Heart Association*, researchers discovered that women who closely followed the DASH diet were 31 percent less likely to develop cardiovascular problems.[14] The National Institutes of Health has a helpful guide to lowering your blood pressure that includes a detailed breakdown of the DASH eating plan. You can download a copy at https://www.nhlbi.nih.gov/files/docs/public/heart/hbp_low.pdf.

Remember, consult your healthcare professional before beginning any new eating plan to make sure that it makes sense for you—and for your heart health.

Mediterranean Diet

The principles of the Mediterranean diet are backed by evidenced-based research; it has long been touted as the preferred dietary approach to reducing cardiovascular risk factors. Numerous studies have shown beneficial heart health effects, including lowering LDL-C (bad cholesterol) levels, reducing risk of secondary heart attacks for those who have previously suffered a cardiac event, and an overall reduced risk of cardiovascular mortality.

Keep in mind that the Mediterranean diet, despite its name, is not a diet. Instead, it's a way of eating and living that mimics healthy habits from various countries surrounding the Mediterranean. The foundation of the diet includes cooking more wholesome foods at

---

14   "These diets helped women with diabetes cut heart attack, stroke risk," American Heart Association, September 19, 2019, https://www.heart.org/en/news/2019/09/19/these-diets-helped-women-with-diabetes-cut-heart-attack-stroke-risk.

home; eating more fruits, vegetables, whole grains, legumes, nuts, and seeds; limiting red meat to no more than twice per month; and eating more fish (at least two days per week). The Mediterranean diet also includes eggs and dairy and replaces saturated fats with healthy monounsaturated fats from olive oil.

Both the Mediterranean diet and the DASH diet recommend similar servings of whole grains, fruits, and vegetables per day. However, the Mediterranean diet recommends limiting red meat to only one or two servings per month while encouraging daily consumption of nuts and using olive oil to prepare foods.

This week, we'll spend time on many of the healthy principles central to both the Mediterranean diet and the DASH diet, along with a few other helpful tips we can't wait to share.

EATING HEALTHY AT EVERY MEAL: SIX TIPS FOR SUCCESS

Tip #1: Read It Before You Eat It!
Knowledge is power. To make healthy choices, you need to know what is in the food you are selecting. It begins by reading those labels. When food shopping, don't rely on attractive packaging or the use of the word "healthy" or "natural" in the name. Be heart smart and food wise; look at the "Nutrition Facts" label and ingredients list on the back to decide if this food meets your new, healthy goals.

First, read the "Nutrition Facts" panel to learn how many grams of fat, sugar, and sodium are in the products you're considering. Pay careful attention to the serving size—it is not always the same from one brand to the next. Second, read the ingredients list—they'll be listed in order from largest volume to least. If there is a word you cannot pronounce, it's likely to be a food preservative or chemical additive.

You also want to be on the lookout for key ingredients you'll want to avoid—things like high-fructose corn syrup, partially hydrogenated oil, sugar, and preservatives. A general rule: Foods that have five or fewer ingredients listed tend to be less processed.

Tip #2: Cut the Salt, Sugar, and Saturated Fat

Salt is a major cause of high blood pressure and other related heart diseases. We now know that cutting salt in the diet reduces the risk of heart attacks and stroke. This is yet another reason to eliminate processed foods, because one of their major ingredients is what is referred to as hidden salt. Over 80 percent of salt intake is from processed foods. The American Heart Association encourages women to become salt detectives by reading labels and only eating foods with 140 milligrams or less of sodium per serving, and we agree!

Tips for cutting sodium:

- Eat only canned, frozen, or other types of processed foods labeled "reduced sodium," "sodium-free," "no salt added," or "unsalted."

- Read those food labels (see Tip #1!) and eat only foods with total sodium content of 140 milligrams or less per serving. Be mindful of hidden sodium in breads and salad dressings. Note that sodium may also be listed as MSG (monosodium glutamate).

- Eat steamed, grilled, baked, boiled, and broiled foods and keep sauces, dressings, and cheese "on the side." Be sure to make this request when ordering out.

- Eat high-sodium condiments sparingly. These include ketchup, soy, teriyaki, steak and Worcestershire sauces, flavored seasoning salts, pickles, olives, anchovies, and salted tomato and vegetable juices.

- Season food with pepper, garlic, lemon, or herbs and spices instead of salt and salt seasonings. Salt-free seasonings are fine, but some seasoning blends do contain salt, MSG, or salt products, so read the label.

- Check the hot sauce label. The original red Tabasco sauce is low in sodium, but many other hot sauces are not.

- Rinse canned vegetables, beans, and capers well in plain water to remove some of the sodium.

- Limit or eliminate consumption of processed or cured meats, bacon, hot dogs, sausage, bologna, ham, salami, salted nuts, and cheeses.

- Avoid using margarine, because even though it contains less saturated fat than butter and no cholesterol, one tablespoon still averages about 150 milligrams of sodium.

Sugar is purely empty calories with no nutritional value. Eating food and drinking beverages containing large amounts of sugar is directly related to an increased risk of type 2 diabetes, which in turn increases the risk of stroke and coronary artery disease. All sugary drinks and foods are high in calories and tend to be low in vitamins and minerals, so they fill you up quickly but will not leave you satisfied. This will tempt you into eating more than you need.

We do need some sugar in our diet, and sugar does occur naturally in food. For instance, fruit has fructose and milk has lactose, both natural sugars. The problem comes when we (or the food manufacturers) *add* sugar. These days, most of the sugar we eat comes from processed foods, which is another reason not to eat them. Also be aware that fat-free salad dressings, barbecue sauces, flavored yogurt, some jarred spaghetti sauces, granola bars, ketchup, and sweetened cereals all contain added sugar. Be aware, too, that honey and fruit juices are still sugar, and the body reacts to them the same way it does to any sugar.

The American Heart Association recommends that women limit added sugars to no more than one hundred calories per day, which translates into about six teaspoons (twenty-four grams). Be sure to read the "Nutrition Facts" label on products. Every four grams of sugar is equivalent to one teaspoonful of sugar. To put this in perspective, a bar with twenty grams of sugar is equivalent to five teaspoons. Yikes!

Strategies for cutting sugar:

- Don't buy or eat foods that have any type of sugars listed as one of the first four ingredients. Note that sugar is listed in many ways: sucrose, glucose, fructose, maltose, dextrose, corn syrup, high-fructose corn syrup, brown sugar, brown rice syrup, raw sugar, molasses, concentrated fruit juice, and honey, to name just a few.

- If you see high-fructose corn syrup listed in the ingredients list, put it back and choose another product.

- Eliminate all sugar-sweetened drinks. Sugary carbonated drinks are the single largest source of calories in the American diet. One twelve-ounce can of cola contains more than nine teaspoons (thirty-nine grams) of sugar! Other sugary beverages include sweetened iced teas, lemonade, fruit punches, sugar-flavored waters, and coffee beverages with added sugars. Instead drink water, seltzer, or unsweetened teas.

- Eat whole fruits and vegetables instead of drinking them. Fruit and vegetable juices and nectars are high in sugar (and sometimes sodium) and low in fiber and are much less satisfying.

- Eat candy in moderation. If you crave candy, choose dark chocolate and eat a piece or two to satisfy your craving, but stop there. Dark chocolate with 70 percent cacao content or higher has been shown to have some health benefits, but only if eaten in moderation. Make that bar of dark chocolate last a few days.

Over the years, *fats* have developed a reputation that is unfair and unwarranted; the truth is that some fats are actually essential to a healthy diet. In fact, 25 to 35 percent of your daily calories should come from healthy fats. These fats are found in nut butters, vegetable oils, fatty fish, nuts, seeds, and avocados. They help the body absorb certain vitamins and help with appetite control, because eating fats can keep you from feeling hungry and overeating. Good fats are also helpful in preventing heart disease and certain cancers and are anti-inflammatory.

> OVER THE YEARS, FATS HAVE DEVELOPED A REPUTATION THAT IS UNFAIR AND UNWARRANTED; THE TRUTH IS THAT SOME FATS ARE ACTUALLY ESSENTIAL TO A HEALTHY DIET.

However, there are some fats you should limit or avoid eating:

Saturated fat. This fat is a dietary demon because it raises LDL (bad) cholesterol, a major factor in heart disease and stroke. The American Heart Association recommends that saturated fats make up no more than 5 to 6 percent of an adult diet. As we said earlier, you do need to eat some fats to live, but they should be in the form of monounsaturated or polyunsaturated fats.

Tips for cutting saturated fat:

- Eat only lean cuts of beef, lamb, pork, and poultry without skin and trim as much visible fat as you can from all types of meat before cooking.

- Consume only low-fat (1 percent) or nonfat milk and dairy products.

- Skim the fat off meat-based soups, cooling them in the refrigerator to solidify the fat so that it is easier to remove.

- Substitute canola, avocado, or olive oil or nonstick spray when cooking and sautéing instead of using butter, lard, or bacon grease.

- Steam vegetables or cook them in low-sodium broth or diced tomatoes instead of sautéing or deep-frying.

- Switch to eating soups made from protein-rich legumes, such as kidney beans, black beans, pinto beans, lentils, split peas, and chickpeas, instead of meat.

- Dress your salads with vinegar (or lemon) and heart-healthy cold-pressed extra-virgin olive oil. If using bottled salad dressings, read labels and choose wisely to minimize consumption of fat, sugar, and sodium. When buying a vinaigrette, pour off half of the oil from the bottle, and voilà! You made your own low-fat salad dressing. Remember to also keep salad dressings on the side, dipping your fork into the dressing and then your food.

- Eat plain steamed vegetables or eat them raw dipped in a little low-calorie salad dressing or salsa. You will be surprised how good they taste.

Trans fats. These are the truly bad fats, because they raise LDL (bad) cholesterol and lower HDL (good) cholesterol by making blood platelets stickier. Sticky platelets accelerate the progression of atherosclerosis and increase the risk of heart attack and stroke. Trans fats were unleashed on us by food companies who invented them to make sure their processed snacks, chips, cookies, baked goods, and other foods stayed fresh as long as possible. They did this by taking essentially healthy monounsaturated and polyunsaturated fats and altering them by a process called partial hydrogenation, which makes them solid at room temperature. Because there is no safe limit for trans fats, avoid them, or at least consume them as infrequently as possible. This should be easy, since they are found mostly in snack foods! Although butter is not a trans fat, we still recommend limiting your butter consumption.

One last thing about trans fats: Labels can be misleading! Foods with less than 0.5 grams of trans fat per serving can *legally* claim to be trans fat–free. This means that if you eat more than one serving of a food containing partially hydrogenated oils, you will actually be eating a significant amount of trans fats. If the ingredients list states "partially hydrogenated oil," don't buy it.

Strategies for cutting trans fats:

- Replace the solid fats in your diet—margarine, lard, and shortening—with liquid canola, avocado, or olive oil or use nonstick spray made from healthy oils.

- Top your baked potato with salsa or low-sodium cottage cheese—not butter or margarine.

- Spread your whole-grain toast or English muffins with nut butter or fresh fruit slices or one of the buttery spreads described in the following section—not butter or margarine.

- Bake your own low-fat, low-sugar cakes, cookies, and pastries.

- Limit eating any baked goods and foods made with partially hydrogenated or saturated fats, including pies, doughnuts, crackers, cookies, bars, and french fries.

A Special Note about Margarine, Oil, Butter, and Buttery Spreads

Margarine. Made from vegetable oils and containing no cholesterol, margarine is also higher in "good" fats—polyunsaturated and mono-unsaturated—than butter. But not all margarines are created equal, and some are even unhealthier than butter. This is especially true with hydrogenated margarines (which most are), because they add trans fats.

So when you choose a margarine, a good rule to remember is that the "harder" or more solid the margarine, the more trans fats it contains. Always choose tub varieties over solid sticks.

Liquid vegetable oils. Throw away the lard and bacon fat and use only healthy oils like avocado, canola, corn, safflower, soybean, and olive oil for cooking. These add no more than two grams of saturated fat per tablespoon.

Butter. Butter is made from milk, which comes from animals, and that means that, like meat, it can clog arteries and affect heart health. You should limit butter in your diet and only use whipped, but that doesn't mean you have to miss the taste. There are healthy substitutes.

Buttery spreads. There are now a variety of plant-based spreads in the dairy case alongside the butter and margarine. Read labels carefully, avoiding those high in saturated fats. Some spreads contain phytosterols, a natural plant compound that may reduce LDL (bad) cholesterol when eaten in recommended amounts and as part of a heart-healthy diet. The spreads also taste good and can also be used in cooking and baking.

Tip #3: Eat a Wide Variety of Plant-Based Whole
Foods and Add Color to Your Plate
Fruits, vegetables, grains, and legumes tend to be low in fat and cholesterol, in addition to being excellent sources of fiber, complex car-

bohydrates, vitamins, and minerals. Nuts and seeds are also nutritious plant-based foods that are high in fiber, vitamins, minerals, protein, and healthy fats. These plant-based foods should be the primary staples in your diet (this also reflects the key recommendations of the Mediterranean and DASH diets). Don't forget, however, that the amount of nutrition you get from these plant-based foods depends on how they are cooked. Frying any vegetable, for example, turns a healthy food into an unhealthy one.

When preparing your dinner, make sure most of your plate is devoted to plant-based foods. You should see colors on your plate from fruits and vegetables. Remember that brown rice is better than white, whole grains are better than refined, lightly steamed veggies are better than mushy ones, and green salads are always a healthy choice (as long as you go easy on the dressing).

Another benefit of these foods is that they are all high in fiber—also known as roughage—which is good for your digestive tract, and eating them naturally helps lower blood cholesterol levels. Fiber is the part of the plant that cannot be digested, but it absorbs many times its weight in water, resulting in softer, bulkier stools. A high-fiber diet keeps food moving through the system and keeps you feeling fuller with much less food. Fibrous food also takes longer to chew and slows down the pace of eating. The slower you eat, the less you eat, because it takes time for the brain to get the message from the stomach that it is full. Although it's always important to drink enough water, it's doubly important when eating foods high in fiber to prevent constipation.

Because fiber is so important for a healthy diet, let's spend a little time learning more about it. There are two types of fiber, soluble and insoluble:

- *Soluble fiber.* This type of fiber is partially broken down in water and can actually help lower cholesterol. Oatmeal, oat bran, barley, nuts, seeds, legumes (such as all dried beans and lentils), and fruits contain soluble fiber. A simple step: Pass up the orange, grapefruit, tomato, and other juices and eat the whole vegetable or fruit instead. (Note: Grapefruit has many food-drug interactions with cardiac medications. Check with your pharmacist if you take prescription drugs.)

- *Insoluble fiber.* This type of fiber cannot be broken down in water and does not lower cholesterol, but it is still important to your diet, as it promotes normal bowel function. Whole grains, such as those found in whole wheat bread, brown rice, and bulgur, or any grain that hasn't had its bran and germ removed by milling, all contain insoluble fiber and are also a great source of nutrients.

Many vegetables also contain insoluble fiber. Fresh or frozen carrots, zucchini, celery, tomatoes, broccoli, pumpkin, squash, cucumbers, cabbage, brussels sprouts, turnips, and cauliflower are good choices. Try to stay away from canned vegetables, especially if you have high blood pressure, because of the amount of sodium they contain. If this isn't possible, buy the low-sodium brand or rinse well before heating.

When it comes to packaged grains, read the label and look for main ingredients listed as whole wheat, whole oats, whole rye, or some other whole grain. If the label doesn't specifically say whole grain or says, "made with wheat, oat, or other enriched grain flour," do not buy it.

Curious to know how much you should eat a day? A registered dietitian or your doctor can help you determine how many portions of fruit and vegetables are right for you, but here are some daily guidelines: as part of a total 1,800-calorie diet, eat two cups of fruit, two and one-half cups of vegetables, and six whole-grain products (such as pasta, rice, quinoa, cereal, whole wheat couscous, or a slice of whole-grain bread) per day. Based on recommendations from the Institute of Medicine, daily fiber goals for women fifty and younger are twenty-five grams per day and twenty-one grams for women fifty and older.[15]

Tip #4: Eat at Home More Often and Cut
Back on Eating Processed Foods

We've talked a lot about the health risks of eating ultraprocessed foods. Let's take a minute to understand the difference. Unprocessed foods are whole foods in their natural state, like fruits, vegetables, whole grains, dried beans, peas, nuts, and seeds. With these foods, the vitamins, minerals, and nutrients are intact. All other foods have some degree of processing, but not all processed foods are bad. For example, a high-fiber, whole-grain breakfast cereal is processed and still a good heart-healthy choice. What we want you to focus on is reducing or eliminating the ultraprocessed foods from your lifestyle—foods with added sodium, sugar, fats, additives, preservatives, and artificial colors and flavors. All of the ultraprocessed foods previously mentioned in this book are examples.

There are a few easy and simple tips you can use to make sure that your food choices are as heart-healthy as possible:

- Eat home-cooked meals as often as you can. You will control the quality and quantity of the ingredients—home-cooked meals tend to be lower in calories, sugar, fat, and sodium.

- When food shopping, spend most of your time in the perimeter of the store. This is where the unprocessed foods

---

15   "Report Offers New Eating and Physical Activity Targets to Reduce Chronic Disease Risk," The National Academies of Sciences, Engineering, and Medicine, September 5, 2002, https://www.nationalacademies.org/news/2002/09/report-offers-new-eating-and-physical-activity-targets-to-reduce-chronic-disease-risk.

are located. And the majority of your time should be spent in the produce section. The processed items tend to be stocked in a store's middle aisles.

- Remember, if you buy it, chances are you will eat it. Our motto is "Don't buy it. Can't eat it!"

- Put your fork down between bites to encourage yourself to eat more slowly and mindfully.

- Cut down on eating heavily processed foods. In Week 1, we encouraged you to choose pantry staples that are less processed, things like sprouted or whole-grain breads, pastas, and cereals, beans, fruits, and vegetables. Cook what you can from scratch and buy the healthiest versions of those you are unable to cook yourself.

- Make eating enjoyable. Share meals with friends and family. If you have children living at home, try to get everyone together for a meal as often as you can—and leave the cell phones in another room! Human interaction is also good for your health.

- Don't forget to hydrate! Drinking any type of nonalcoholic beverage, especially water, seltzer, and other nonsweetened beverages, is important to keep the organs running smoothly and to prevent dehydration.

- Eat a variety of foods. Variety really is the spice of life, so change it up! Choose different-color fruits and vegetables to eat each week. Different colors offer different vitamins, minerals, and antioxidants. This also sets a good example for the young ones in your life to be exposed to different foods and tastes.

- Eat slowly, chew your food well, and stop when you are full. It's OK to leave food on your plate.

- Eat well-balanced meals. Include whole grains, protein, fruits, and vegetables.

- Choose healthy snacks. When you need a snack, choose a piece of fruit paired with a handful of almonds over that doughnut you hear calling your name!

- Take home-prepared meals and snacks with you to work to avoid the spontaneous need to purchase unhealthy convenience items if you get hungry.

Tip #5: Institute Meatless Mondays and Eat Fish Two Times a Week
The "meatless Mondays" movement is an easy way to help cut down on eating high-fat protein (like red meat), boost your intake of antioxidant- and fiber-rich plant-based foods, and begin getting accustomed to eating more plant-based meals. Simply eliminate meat from your meals one day each week and, over time, continue to reduce red meat so that you are eating it only a few times per month, as supported by the Mediterranean diet. Learning to go "meatless" will help you expand your cooking repertoire so that you may eventually be able to cook more adventurous and tastier no-meat meals.

If you're not one who enjoys vegetarian dining, eating fish is a great way to get the benefits of protein without adding saturated fat and cholesterol to your diet. Fish is also high in omega-3 polyunsaturated fatty acids, which greatly reduces the risk of developing coronary artery disease. Omega-3s help decrease cardiac arrhythmia, lower triglyceride levels, slow the buildup of plaque in arteries, and slightly lower blood pressure. All fish contain this healthy fat, but salmon, mackerel, sardines, trout, bluefish, albacore tuna, and herring are especially rich in omega-3s. The American Heart Association recommends eating at least two three-ounce servings of these types of fish each week in order to reap the health benefits.

Again, as with vegetables, frying destroys the health benefits of fish, as does adding creamy sauces. Grill, bake, broil, or poach fish. Add a little olive oil and season with lemon and garlic (before or after cooking) for a simple, delicious, and healthy meal.

Tip #6: Skip the Second Helpings

It doesn't matter how healthy your diet is; if you eat too much you will gain weight. Controlling portion sizes is a vital part of weight management.

It's easier to overeat these days, because portion sizes have gotten larger over the years. For example, in the 1970s, soda was sold in eight-ounce bottles. As time went on, the portion size increased to twelve ounces and then was "supersized" to twenty ounces, an increase of over 145 calories! In 1990, an average bagel was three inches in diameter (approximately 145 calories). Today's average bagel is five to six inches in diameter (approximately 350 calories), more than double the original in calories—and that's without the toppings. Even plates and bowls have gotten bigger. The problem is that these big portions now seem normal.

But you can take charge and take control of your portion sizes. When you eat at home, we recommend using a nine-inch plate. Fill half of your plate with vegetables, one-quarter with protein, and one-quarter with a whole-grain carbohydrate like quinoa, brown rice, or even a sweet potato. Once you've prepared your plate, decide that the meal you've prepared is exactly what you'll need; try to avoid returning for a second helping. When dining out, eat only what you know to be a sensible portion and then push the rest to the side of your plate.

Restaurant portions are almost always excessive. Ask for a container to take the rest home. You'll have a meal for another day.

Spend some time paying attention to the size of your meals and also to the space taken up on your plate by each type of food. That way, you won't need a scale or calorie counter. Later in the book, we'll share some easy and fun ways to "eyeball" healthy portions of various foods. These tips will help you to portion out your meals at home and eat less when dining out. Learning to reduce the volume of food you typically eat takes repetition and time to adjust. Remember to use smaller plates and bowls and to put the food away to help avoid those second helpings.

HEALTHY SWAPS

We have great news: you can enjoy the tastes you love *and* eat a healthy diet. What you've eaten in the past may have caused health problems, but there is no reason you cannot enjoy the same tastes in healthier versions. It's simply a matter of making a few thoughtful swaps.

The chart below shows just how easy it is. You'll find many delicious and satisfying substitutes for the foods you enjoy. Even though some of these substitutions may not taste exactly the same at first, give yourself the time and the space to get accustomed to these slightly different tastes. In this chapter we've already suggested healthier alternatives for some foods, but here are some additional suggestions.

> YOU CAN ENJOY THE TASTES YOU LOVE *AND* EAT A HEALTHY DIET.

INSTEAD OF ...	TRY ...
Full-fat soft and whole-milk cheeses (e.g., Colby, cheddar, brie, pimento and packaged processed spreads or presliced processed cheese slices)	Nonfat, reduced-fat, or vegetarian varieties
Full-fat and sugar-filled dairy products (milk, ice cream, yogurt, cottage cheese, cream cheese, sour cream)	Nonfat, low-fat, or nondairy alternative products (0 percent Greek yogurt is a great substitute for sour cream and mayo)
Farina, grits, or sugar-sweetened oatmeal	Regular or steel-cut plain oatmeal (not instant), quinoa, or millet
Premade salad dressing	Homemade dressing with extra-virgin olive oil and vinegar or lemon juice and herbs
White potatoes, mashed potatoes	Sweet potatoes, mashed cauliflower, or root vegetables like parsnips
White rice	Brown whole-grain or wild rice, cauliflower rice, or quinoa
Refined white bread, pasta, flour	Whole-grain or sprouted-grain breads, whole-grain pastas (quinoa, brown rice, chickpea or red lentil pasta), zucchini noodles, spaghetti squash

INSTEAD OF ...	TRY ...
Sugary, low-fiber cereals	Bran or whole-grain, low-sugar cereals, >5g fiber
White sugar	Natural sugar substitutes in moderation Reduce the amount of sugar you bake and cook with, substituting with fruit instead (i.e., dates, natural applesauce, prunes)
Soda (including diet), fruit juice, nectars	Plain, sparkling, or flavored water or unsweetened iced tea
Pasta, couscous	Whole wheat, quinoa, or lentil-based varieties, zucchini noodles and spaghetti squash or whole wheat couscous
Salted nuts and seeds	Raw nuts and seeds (almonds, cashews, pecans, hazelnuts, walnuts, Brazil nuts, sunflower, hemp, pumpkin ...)
Fatty cuts of beef and pork (porterhouse, rib eye, pork shoulder, spare ribs)	Fish, skinless chicken or turkey breast, tofu, beans, or very lean cuts of beef or pork (round or loin cuts)
Butter	Olive oil (great on whole-grain toast), extra-virgin olive oil

Use this new skill of making healthy swaps when dining out too. Don't want the fries? Ask to substitute a vegetable, side salad, or baked potato instead. Don't want the rice? Ask for a double helping of vegetables. Don't want fried chicken cutlet? Ask if grilled chicken can be substituted. Instead of a hamburger, try a chicken or turkey burger. We'll cover dining out more specifically later in this chapter.

YOUR WEEKLY CHALLENGE

This week, commit to making some heart-healthy changes in how you eat, how much you eat, and what you eat. Use this checklist to get started, and add new goals as you check these off.

My goal(s) for this week:

☐ Try a Meatless Monday.
☐ Eat fish twice a week.
☐ Try a new vegetable.
☐ Experiment with a healthy swap.
☐ Replace a takeout meal with one I make myself.

Part Two: Healthy Eating at Home and Dining Out

Now let's put your food knowledge into practice. Some rules will differ when you are dining out because you may need to think on your feet and make substitutions for what is available on the menu. Preparation is key: restaurant eating presents more of a challenge than cooking for yourself. Some of what you read in this chapter will reinforce what you learned in earlier chapters, as some rules bear repeating. Are you ready?

PRESENTING YOUR NEW PLATE!

Whether you are eating at home or in a restaurant, this is what your plate should look like. This simple graphic was designed by the USDA to remind Americans how easy it is to eat healthfully. So from now on, this is all you need to know to balance your food choices and avoid overly large portions.

- **Half the plate** is filled with fruits and vegetables. The proportion of each is up to you. Just make sure your selections take up half the plate.

- **One-quarter of the plate** is filled with lean protein—lean meat, skinless chicken, fish or tofu or plant-based protein.

- **One-quarter of the plate** contains sweet potatoes, brown rice, or whole grains.

- **The eight-ounce cup** or glass contains water, low-fat milk, sparkling or flavored water, unsweetened iced tea, or some other nonsugary, no-calorie beverage.

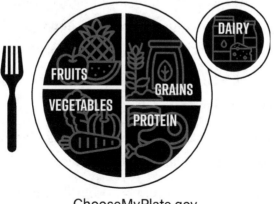

ChooseMyPlate.gov

SERVING SIZES

We use the illustration of the plate because it's a clear and easy way to think about healthy eating. But dinner plates can vary in size, making it difficult to determine an appropriate portion size. In part three of this book, we'll share more specific information on how much of each food is considered a healthy serving.

HEALTHY COOKING SUGGESTIONS

Now that you know the types and quantities of foods that you are going to eat, here are some suggestions for cooking that food in ways that won't add sugar, salt, fat, and calories:

- Grill, bake, roast, broil, and poach foods rather than frying or sautéing.

- Add flavor with garlic, lemon juice, herbs, and spices as a substitute for salt.

- Don't forget the pepper. Black pepper, hot pepper (sauce, fresh, or ground), smoked paprika, and chilies all add flavor and, depending on the pepper, a new dimension of heat.

- Limit meals with meat and poultry, and eat fish at least twice a week and vegetarian at least once a week (Meatless Mondays). Try turning your favorite meat dishes into vegetarian versions, such as vegetable lasagna, chili, or pasta sauce.

- Use a rack when roasting poultry or meat so it doesn't sit in its own drippings.

- Don't baste meat or poultry with drippings. Instead use wine, low-salt stock, or tomato or lemon juice.

- Grill or roast vegetables to bring out their natural sugars. Be careful not to overcook. Cut them to a uniform size, toss with one tablespoon of olive oil per cup of vegetables, and roast on a cookie sheet or on the grill until tender.

- Use avocado, olive, and canola oil for cooking, and extra-virgin olive oil, flax oil, and walnut oils for dressings and marinades.

- Add unsalted nuts (almonds, walnuts, hazelnuts, pecans, cashews, pistachios, etc.) to your daily diet by eating a handful or sprinkling them chopped or whole over salads, pasta, and vegetables.

- Creatively add vegetables to meals and snacks. Add chopped vegetables to omelets and fruit smoothies, eat salads for lunch and dinner, and pile sandwiches with cucumber slices, leafy greens, pepper rings, onion slices, and tomatoes.

PLAN AHEAD

Cooking and eating most of your meals at home (and packing a healthy lunch for work) require preparation and planning ahead. This is a great opportunity to get organized, to use the shopping lists we provided earlier, and to keep them updated with new foods you want to try and staples you need to replace. In addition, these suggestions can help you get dinner on the table with a minimum of fuss:

Cook your favorite foods. Find healthy meals that you like, and make them the basis of your weekly meals. If you are dealing with an old family favorite, chances are it needs to be updated. Those traditional recipes tend to be high in salt, sugar, and fat, so update them for your new, healthy lifestyle. Get creative.

Buy a new cookbook. There are lots of great cookbooks that focus on health. Get one and add a few new dishes to your menu—it'll be like trying out a new restaurant.

Cook ahead. Either set aside time at the beginning of the week or use any time you can find to cook more than one meal. That way, all you have to do is heat and serve. Many dishes (like chili, stews, and soups) are even better a day or two after they are made.

Prep your meals. For meals that can't be made ahead, at least peel and cut up the vegetables, skin and/or debone the poultry, marinate meat or fish, or precook what you can. Having part of the meal prepared means more time in the evening to relax.

Make double and freeze one. This works especially well when making a pasta sauce, soup, or casserole. Thaw frozen meals in the fridge for 12 to 24 hours before you cook or reheat them.

Precut vegetables (and fruit) for snacks. Carrots, celery, cucumbers, steamed broccoli, asparagus, and apples are all good. Use hummus, smashed avocado, or salsa as a dip.

HOW NOT TO OVEREAT AT HOME

Overeating can be an issue if you live alone (or eat alone). You may find it helpful and fun to invite friends over to join you or gather the family or your significant other at the dinner table. But even with people around, it's easy to sneak in that extra mouthful or to snack while cleaning up. Beware of these pitfalls when eating at home:

Limit alcohol. Limit alcohol to one five-ounce glass of red wine (or less) *per day.*

Don't "sample" while cooking. A small taste to adjust seasonings is fine, but excessive tasting or snacking while cooking can seriously increase the number of calories you consume.

Don't "pick" while cleaning up. Same reason as above!

Eat only what is on your plate and do not go back for seconds. Keep the serving dishes off the table. Better yet, serve the food directly from the cooking pots. Pack up what is left in the pots for another meal.

Use smaller plates and bowls. It may surprise you, but this really works! Today's plates are much larger than the ones we used in the mid-twentieth century. The average American plate is twelve inches wide. That's three inches larger than we recommend. If your plates are oversize, buy some eight- or nine-inch plates on sale or at a thrift store. Or use a "salad" plate as your dinner plate.

Eat slowly. This is why it's good to have company. Talking makes the meal go more slowly. It takes time for your brain to catch up with your stomach. You can be full, but your brain won't receive the message if you eat too fast.

Stop when you are full. If you aren't able to finish your meal, don't force yourself. You do not need to clear your plate.

Don't watch TV or talk on the phone while eating. Pay attention to your meal. If you are distracted, you won't be totally aware of how much you are eating (another reason to plate the meal in the kitchen).

SNACKING

We understand. From time to time, everyone needs a snack. It is natural to feel hungry a few hours after a meal. The secret is to make sure that you space your meals and snacks evenly throughout the day and avoid constantly grazing or nibbling. If you are always hungry around 3:00 p.m., then take a prepared healthy snack with you to work. Having a healthy go-to snack on hand will help you avoid buying a muffin or sticking your hand in a jar of candy. Be sure to have plenty of healthy options available to help get you through those times when your cravings take center stage! Try these tips:

- Keep snacks to no more than two hundred calories.

- Take your snacks with you to work or in the car if you're out running errands all day.

- Eat balanced snacks, including a carbohydrate and protein or fat source. For example, pair an apple with a one-hundred-calorie snack pack of almonds or spread one tablespoon of natural nut butter on a medium banana. Try a cheese stick with a few whole-grain crackers.

- Use sliced cucumbers, tomatoes, or zucchini as "chips." Top with low-fat cheese or low-salt cottage cheese. Try dipping them in hummus or guacamole.

- Eat a small sweet potato sprinkled with cinnamon. This will be a satisfying midafternoon or evening snack.

- Try three cups of air-popped popcorn sprinkled with parmesan cheese.

- Premeasure all snacks. Since snacking is usually done in front of the TV or while otherwise distracted, don't sit with an open package of any snack food (even if it is a healthy one), because you will lose track of how much you have eaten. Break down packages of snack foods into individually portioned bags. It's also more cost-effective to do it yourself than to buy them premeasured.

DINING OUT

The same rules apply to dining in a restaurant or eating at someone else's house. Once you are not responsible for the preparation of your meal, ingredients and portion size may not be consistent with your new, healthier lifestyle. Here's how to make any meal healthier, even if you don't cook or serve it yourself.

First, let's take a careful look at the challenges. We've broken these down into three major challenges.

THE THREE MAJOR CHALLENGES OF DINING OUT

1	An entire menu—cocktails, appetizers, entrees and desserts—with no limit as to what you can order. And a bottomless breadbasket!
2	Additional calories, salt, fat, and sugar are added to many dishes in the form of sauces, gravies, toppings, and condiments.
3	Portion sizes are generally significantly larger than what your body needs.

Tips for Overcoming the Three Major Dining-Out Challenges

First: If possible, review the menu online before you go to the restaurant. That way, you will not be making choices on the spur of the moment. Decide precisely what you're going to order—and stick to your plan! If that is not possible, take a good look at the menu before you make your selection, looking for the heart-healthy choices that are now part of your daily eating plan. Don't be afraid to ask the server questions, such as how the dish is prepared (since it's not always obvious from the menu). Make substitution requests if needed. As a first step, eliminate the unhealthy foods, such as anything pan- or deep-fried, scalloped (cooked in cream sauce), au gratin (cooked in cheese sauce), or stuffed (you never know every ingredient in stuffing, and the server probably doesn't know, either).

Second: Most restaurants add extra salt to their food, but that doesn't mean that you have to eat it. Be confident as you ask that no salt be added to your food. When you consider your choices, concentrate on anything that is steamed, broiled, baked, grilled, poached, or roasted. But you still need to ask the server if any of these foods are cooked in butter, have butter added, or are served with a sauce, gravy, or a topping. If so, it doesn't mean that you shouldn't order it, but it does mean that you should request that these calorie-laden extras be served "on the side." That way, you can use them sparingly and still enjoy the flavor they provide. Most restaurants are happy to oblige. You can also ask for an extra lemon to add more flavor to your dish, especially for fish or seafood.

Third: If you don't see a selection that meets your new healthy lifestyle, ask them to make you one that does. Requesting broiled fish or chicken is not unreasonable, nor is asking that vegetables be steamed and served without butter or that the potato be baked instead of mashed or fried. Most restaurants will comply with reasonable requests. Besides, we bet you aren't the only diner making them!

Additional Restaurant Recommendations

Tip 1: The buffet! Nothing—we mean nothing—is as dangerous as the restaurant buffet table. The trick to healthy buffet eating is to fill up by eating the healthy foods first, which will leave less room for the dangerous, full-fat, empty-calorie desserts. With buffets you'll need to exert some extra effort to adhere to your healthy eating plan.

Move with purpose as you navigate a buffet:

- Sail past the bread to the salads and fill your plate to the brim with healthy lettuce and vegetables, nuts, and fruit. Top your salad off with minimal dressing or plain vinegar or lemon.

- Try a cup of the tasty soups that are offered, especially the clear or vegetable-based ones, not the creamy ones.

- Choose protein wisely by staying away from all meats, poultry, and fish that are floating in sauce or gravy and opt for those that look as close as possible to what you would prepare for yourself at home.

- Opt for the plain rice, the baked or boiled potatoes, or a tiny plate of pasta. Remember, only a quarter of your plate should be devoted to carbs.

- Select vegetables that aren't swimming in butter. If that isn't possible, have another helping of salad.

- If you must splurge on dessert, eat one, but don't go back for seconds unless it's fresh fruit, which should have been your first choice! Granted, you may have trouble getting past the dessert table, but there's no law against sharing one or eating only half.

Tip 2: Remember the salad option and choose salads wisely. Adding a piece of broiled chicken or fish to a specialty salad is always a good go-to option. This makes for a satisfying meal that fills out your plate perfectly, and it allows you to eat a piece of that delicious restaurant bread. However, read the ingredients carefully; many restaurants add dried fruit, bacon, marinated vegetables, pasta, and other cured meats to their meal-size salads. Even smaller dinner salads can arrive dressed up with bacon bits—an ingredient you're better off not eating. Always ask what is in the salad so you are not surprised. Only use the house vinaigrette if it is prepared with olive oil, and be sure to ask for the dressing on the side so you can control how much of it you eat—or dress your salad with vinegar or lemon juice.

Tip 3: Tiptoe through the appetizer minefield. Appetizers are especially dangerous since you are usually hungry when you get to the restaurant; many appetizers sound delicious. It's the same principle as going food shopping when you're hungry.

Looking over a menu of appetizers on an empty stomach is never a good idea—you will want them all! One way around this is to eat a small snack before you leave for the restaurant, such as a piece of fruit or some raw vegetables to avoid being overly hungry. This will take the edge off your appetite. It is very hard to make a healthy decision when you are starving! Most appetizers are fried or loaded with cheese, heavy sauces, and dressings. To avoid blowing your calorie budget with an appetizer, try starting your meal with a simple salad or a vegetable-based soup—not one made with cream (hint: not Caesar salad).

Tip 4: Check menus for "healthy" symbols. Many restaurants today are trying to accommodate patrons who are looking for simpler, healthier dishes. These are noted (sometimes with their calorie counts and other nutritional information) right on the menu. Check out the restaurant's website ahead of time to see if they offer healthier choices on the menu, and whenever possible choose restaurants that offer healthier, lighter foods.

Tip 5: Make substitutions. Remember how you made healthy swaps at home? You can do the same thing when dining out. In place of fried items or refined white carbs, ask to substitute brown rice for white rice or a baked potato, vegetable, or salad in place of French fries. Request a side of vegetables instead of a side of pasta, grilled chicken in place of a fried cutlet, or a chicken or turkey burger in place of a beef burger (maybe even a lettuce wrap instead of a bun). We understand that occasionally you may want to splurge on a steak. This is OK if done occasionally. Be sure to choose a lean cut like filet mignon or sirloin and request no butter be added to your meat. You get the idea. Make your restaurant meal fit your new healthy ideals.

Tip 6: Share your meal or take half home. Restaurant portions are generally larger than what is recommended as a healthy serving size. Some places charge a fee for sharing a dish, but it may be worth it. If you don't want to pay extra, take the other half home to enjoy for lunch or dinner the next day.

Tip 7: Don't worry about getting your money's worth. Thinking this way could be your downfall. Eating out is about being with people and having a good time. If it's value you want, you'll get that with home-cooked meals. Eating in is good for the pocketbook, but eating out with friends is good for the soul!

Tip 8: If you slip up, don't despair! When you do eat out, try to be extra vigilant, but if you do slip up, simply be sure to eat healthy the rest of the day or the next day.

Tip 9: Don't pass up the wine. If you drink, feel free to have a glass of red wine with dinner—but make it your only glass of the day. Otherwise, stick to still or sparkling water and lemon or unsweetened iced tea.

Tip 10: Yes, you can have dessert. A decaffeinated cappuccino or a cup of hot tea, especially green tea, can double as a dessert, and fresh fruit is always a sweet and perfect end to a good meal. Opt to order one dessert for every four to six people at the table, so everyone gets a forkful of delicious pie or cake or a spoonful (or maybe two) of ice cream. If there are only two of you dining, stick with the coffee and fruit, unless you're able to leave some of the dessert on the plate!

HOLIDAY EATING

There's no doubt about it, holidays (especially those that focus on food) are a bit more challenging when you're trying to control what you eat. Holidays are especially challenging, because so many foods we associate with celebrations are filled with the very ingredients we are working to avoid. For some of us, there may be the added stress and tension of dealing with relatives. It's easy to revert back to old habits and lose yourself in food, especially when holiday dishes are probably childhood favorites and relatives are making sure you taste every one of them.

Be it Thanksgiving, Christmas, a Passover seder or a Fourth of July barbecue, many of the holiday foods are abundant in calories. But if you apply the rules you learned earlier in this book and in this chapter, you will get through the holidays without a problem.

Exercise can fall to the bottom of the list during holidays. If that happens, you won't be burning as many calories as usual. If possible, try to add additional steps to your day, or sneak in an extra exercise class. If that is not possible, be extra vigilant when it comes to portion size. Eat less now; work less later.

If you are the cook, make this the time to prepare old favorites in healthier ways, cut down on the sugar, reduce the fat and salt, use the cooking techniques we talked about earlier, and make sure there's a big salad and lots of vegetables on the menu!

If it's potluck, this is your chance to bring a healthy dish that you know you can eat.

Above all, the holidays are for enjoying the company of your family and friends. You may not lose weight during this time, but stay as active as you can because that will decrease your appetite, lower your stress, and increase your metabolism. Your holiday goal is not to lose weight—it's not to gain any!

> **YOUR HOLIDAY GOAL IS NOT TO LOSE WEIGHT— IT'S NOT TO GAIN ANY!**

VACATIONS

When it comes to maintaining a healthy eating and exercise plan, vacations can also be challenging, especially if every meal is a restaurant meal. Even if you spend your vacation visiting friends, you may be eating out a lot or tempted with special meals and treats that your host prepared especially for you. Remember, you have made great progress with each week, and you've learned how the choices you make are helping you to feel healthier and more energetic. When you're away from home, you can continue to choose heart-healthy foods, and avoid those that are not.

Everything you've learned about healthy eating and dining out applies to eating on vacation, so we won't repeat it here. But the main rule to remember is that being on vacation is no reason to ignore healthy eating habits. You don't want to undo weeks or months of effort in just a week or two! We do want to share some techniques and advice that you can use to avoid the pitfalls you'll encounter when traveling.

Road Trips

When you're traveling by car, avoid fast-food restaurants. Pack a cooler of sandwiches, beverages, and healthy snacks and picnic along the way. Remember to take a short walk before getting back in the car. Save your food stops for those great farm stands and choose lots of regional fruits and vegetables that are delicious to eat raw. Don't forget to stay hydrated—water is always a good choice.

Many of the same rules apply when you're traveling by plane, train, or bus. Pack your own meals and snacks. Take time to stretch and walk up and down the aisles whenever it is safe to do so.

If you run out of food and must eat out, you know what to do, and if you don't, then reread this chapter!

FOODS AND SNACKS THAT TRAVEL WELL

Traveling presents special problems, because the available foods may not be the healthiest choices. But you can take charge by packing a few snacks that travel well so that you always have plenty of healthy choices.

When you're getting ready for a road trip, make sure that you pack a few of these tasty, healthy, and energizing "travel" foods:

- Peanut (or other nut—no added sugar or salt) butter sandwiches (try adding banana and apple slices, all-natural fruit spread or smashed strawberries for natural sweetness) or pumpkin seeds

- Individually portioned unsalted nuts and seeds

- Carrot sticks with individually packaged hummus or salsa

- Plain popcorn

- Cheese sticks with whole-grain crackers

- Fruit: Apples, peaches, bananas, clementines, oranges or grapes ... fruit is the perfect road trip food! Don't forget to pair with some unsalted nuts.

When You Arrive at Your Destination

If you are staying in a hotel, your room will probably have a refrigerator, and if you are diabetic, most establishments will supply you with a small fridge for insulin storage if you request one; this will also give you safe storage for food and snacks. If not, you can keep food in your cooler or insulated bag and use the hotel's ice machine to keep foods cool.

Take inventory of the snack foods you have left and restock with items like fresh fruit, yogurt, cheese, nuts, whole-grain bread and nut butter, or whole-grain cereal and nonfat milk.

Breakfast on the Go

THE BREAKFAST BUFFET

Breakfast buffets present a challenge because they are loaded with foods, each of which could constitute a breakfast on its own or shouldn't be served at breakfast at all (like doughnuts). Our advice is to sample a few things that you wouldn't ordinarily eat at home, but the key word is "sample." One breakfast buffet slice of bacon or sausage won't jeopardize your health, but we understand the difficulty of being confronted with many selections and not being able to enjoy them all. Try a few of these strategies for making wise choices that will leave you feeling satisfied and not deprived:

- Eggs are always a good choice, including vegetable omelets (no cheese), ready-made scrambled, soft-boiled, hard-boiled, or poached (skip the fried eggs).

- One slice of bacon, a small piece of ham, or one link or sausage patty is fine.

- Oatmeal or bran cereal (with low-fat or fat-free milk) is always a good choice.

- Fresh fruit can be used to top your cereal or as a breakfast "dessert."

- English muffin with peanut butter.

- One small whole wheat roll, slice of bread, or bran muffin is fine, but avoid the Danish, bagels, doughnuts, scones, and biscuits.

THE FAST-FOOD BREAKFAST

Ordering in a restaurant or diner gives you the latitude to get a breakfast that resembles what you would make for yourself at home, but fast-food establishments don't fit that bill. You will need to order within their menu. Some fast-food places do offer egg-white sandwiches cooked to order. At other places you may be able to order an egg on an English muffin or breakfast burrito. Ask for no bacon, sausage, ham, or home fries. If oatmeal is on the menu, be sure it's not presweetened or loaded with dried fruit and nuts (ask if you can add them yourself).

BEVERAGES

Coffee and tea (hot or iced) are OK with milk and no or minimal sweetener.

Stay away from high-calorie, low-fiber juice, even if it comes with your meal. It's not worth it in terms of your health. You're better off drinking water.

Happy travels!

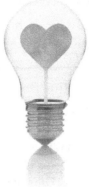

Week 4

P: PARTNER WITH YOUR DOCTOR, FAMILY, AND FRIENDS

Partnerships are powerful. They impact every facet of our lives and have the potential to increase performance, perseverance, and results. When it comes to being heart-healthy, partnerships are extra important.

As you begin Week 4 of the Six S.T.E.P.S. in Six Weeks Program, you have already restocked your kitchen with healthy foods, you are choosing to move more every day, and you are enjoying colorful plates of fruits and vegetables and better managing your relationship with salt and sugar. Now it's time to consider the importance of partnerships on your journey to heart health.

We will start with finding a doctor you like and trust. How pleased are you with your current doctor, and how trusting are you? Your relationship with your doctor is of utmost importance in your quest to stay healthy and free of heart disease. Think of your doctor as your partner in health; like any successful partnership, this one needs a bond of trust and an open line of communication.

The Power of the Patient/ Healthcare Team Bond

When was the last time you saw your doctor?[16] If you only go to the doctor when you are sick, we need you to rethink that strategy. We know—you're busy. Your schedule is already full. It's easy to put off making a doctor's appointment because of the demands of your job and your family and other responsibilities. And far too often, women schedule regular doctor visits for everyone but themselves.

We want to challenge you to rethink those priorities. Part of becoming heart smarter is choosing to prioritize your health. Remember that many people who suffer fatal heart attacks didn't even know they had heart disease. The best way to diagnose and treat heart problems and the medical issues that lead to heart attack is to be seen regularly by a doctor.

YOUR ANNUAL WELL-WOMAN VISIT

Any good partnership depends on your willingness to invest time in building that relationship. The way to forge a true partnership with your physician is through an annual well-woman visit. This provides you with an opportunity to review your health concerns with your doctor, and it provides your doctor with an opportunity to learn about you and your family history and recent changes

---

16   Some individuals may receive primary healthcare services from another healthcare professional, such as a nurse practitioner. The important point is that you have a relationship with a primary healthcare provider.

in your health status, as well as to perform or discuss with you appropriate screening measures. At your well-woman visit, your doctor will examine you for any signs of heart disease, and he or she will recommend steps you can take to reduce risk factors before complications arise. This may include cholesterol screening, blood pressure monitoring, body mass index assessment, and other evaluations specifically designed to help assess your heart health. It is a great way to help lower your risk of heart attack or stroke, and also to give you some peace of mind.

The well-woman visit also allows your doctor to review and identify any other health concerns and to ensure that you have received necessary and appropriate preventive measures, such as flu, tetanus, and pneumonia shots. At this visit, your doctor will evaluate your health needs based on several factors, including your age, family history, and past health history, and may also recommend that you be screened for other health issues that are unique to or more prevalent in women, including mammograms for breast cancer, Pap smears for cervical cancer, prenatal care, and bone-mass measurements for osteoporosis, as well as gender-neutral screenings and services such as colon cancer screening, obesity screening, and counseling and screening for behavioral health concerns.

Because so many women routinely schedule visits to obstetricians and gynecologists, these healthcare professionals are a valuable resource with whom you can discuss things like nutrition, weight, exercise programs, and even sleep and stress. Don't be afraid to ask questions about all areas of your wellness—including your cardiovascular health—when you're meeting with your gynecologist or obstetrician. It's also important to note that more specialized care is optimal as you near menopause—an internist or family practitioner will be a valuable ally to support your goals for healthy living.

Just as you prepared for each of the lifestyle changes outlined in the previous chapters, you need to get into the mindset of scheduling a yearly well-woman visit. If you are anxious about going to the doctor for any reason, a yearly checkup should help put those fears to rest because they can validate the positive changes you are making. What's more, a yearly well-woman visit can diagnose potential problems before they become serious.

If you still have doubts about the need for an annual well-woman visit, those of you with children will recall well-baby visits to the pediatrician. You took them to the doctor just to make sure everything was fine, because you cared about their health and well-being. We all see the dentist for regular checkups and cleaning, even if we don't have a toothache, in order to keep our teeth and gums healthy. We see the gynecologist for a Pap smear or to schedule a mammogram. So it makes sense to add your medical doctor or internist to your schedule of annual visits. Early detection and treatment of many types of medical problems, including heart disease, saves lives.

FINDING A DOCTOR

If you don't have a primary care clinician, now is the time to find one you like and trust. An emergency room visit is not a substitute for an annual physical. You need to partner with a doctor who will get to know you and your health history. To help, here are a few suggestions and guidelines to make your search easier:

- Ask family, friends, and coworkers for a recommendation and make a list.

- Check the listing of participating physicians on your health insurance plan's website to see if any are on your recommended list.

- Be sure the physician accepts your insurance when you make the appointment. If you don't have insurance, make that clear when you call.

- Talk to coworkers who have the same insurance plan as you, and ask for the name of their doctor and if they have had a positive experience.

- Check the website of a local hospital or health organization to see if they accept your insurance and for a listing of the physicians who work there.

- Consider only physicians who are board-certified (which means they have passed special training and testing requirements) for the specialties of family medicine or general internal medicine.

- Check the physician's office hours and location(s); convenience should play a role in your selection.

- Choose a physician of the sex you will be most comfortable with.

- Take your time and do some research. Finding the right doctor is important to your future health. You are looking for a doctor who will be your partner for a very long time.

IDENTIFYING THE RIGHT HEALTHCARE PARTNER

In order to stay healthy, you need to have a good relationship with your doctor. If you don't like a doctor for *any* reason—be it trust, personality, or something you can't put your finger on—then find another one. When you don't like your doctor, you are less likely to make an appointment to see him or her, so find someone you like and with whom you can establish a trusting relationship. And don't feel guilty if you have decided your doctor is not the right partner for you. It's not your fault. Find someone you trust—someone you feel comfortable asking questions—and don't settle for less, no matter what.

If you do decide to change doctors, remember that your medical records belong to you. Be sure to complete any paperwork necessary to ensure an efficient transfer of records from your former doctor to your new doctor.

MAKING THE MOST OUT OF THE FIRST VISIT

For those of you who are changing doctors or seeing a primary care physician for the first time, you will want to make the most of that first visit. If you are nervous, you are not alone. It's common for patients to be nervous or anxious when seeing a doctor—especially on the first visit. If you would feel more comfortable, consider bringing a family member or friend to this initial visit.

You will want to optimize your time with your new doctor, so here's what you can do to make the most of it:

- Be on time or a few minutes early.

- Have your insurance cards and medical information handy. If you don't have insurance, make sure you have the name of the person you spoke to when you made your appointment.

We've encouraged you to keep a notebook or journal and to prepare your Personal Health Inventory. This is an opportunity to use that valuable resource! As a reminder, here is some of the information you'll want to have ready for your meeting with your healthcare professional:

- Every medication you take, including dosage and time of day taken (be sure to include all over-the-counter medications, including botanicals, vitamins, minerals, aspirin, cold remedies and allergy medication; if you prefer, you can gather up all the bottles, put them in a bag, and bring them with you)

- Your family medical history (make a detailed list of the illnesses that affected your parents, grandparents, aunts, uncles, or siblings; also list first-degree relatives who have passed away and indicate their age and cause of death)

- Any allergies you have to drugs, food, animals, pollen, and so on

- Your detailed medical history, including hospitalizations, surgeries and chronic conditions

- All of your medical complaints: Detailed descriptions of the pain or problem and how long it has bothered you (if, for example, you have felt a stabbing pain in your right arm that moves down to your elbow, write it down and describe it to your doctor in those exact words; don't hide or downplay symptoms—they may be important)

- Questions you want to ask your doctor (see the worksheet included in this chapter for some suggestions)

Use your journal to record everything that the doctor tells you, because it's impossible to remember everything that was said. In addition, *never* be afraid to ask the doctor to repeat information or to explain it again if you didn't understand or hear it the first time.

Your annual checkup tells you so much more than the state of your health at that moment. An annual checkup enables the doctor to diagnose and head off potential problems based on the physical examination in conjunction with your list of concerns and complaints. When you have answers, you will have peace of mind.

QUESTIONS TO ASK YOUR DOCTOR

It's natural to feel nervous before a visit with a healthcare professional, whether in person or by phone. You'll feel more confident if you prepare a list of questions ahead of time. Think about everything you'd like to ask and write it down. You'll want to compile this type of list for *every* doctor's visit.

Here are some suggested questions to get you started. This list is only to be used as a guideline; be sure to personalize it by adding your own questions and concerns.

What is my risk of heart disease based on my evaluation?

_____

_____

_____

When do I schedule my next visit, and is there any further testing to be scheduled before my next visit?

_____

_____

_____

Do I have a cardiovascular condition? How serious is it? What caused it, and how do I best manage it?

_____

_____

_____

What kinds of choices are within my control to favorably impact my condition?

_____

_____

_____

Can any medications prescribed at this visit interact with food or the drugs I already take? What are the possible side effects? Should the medication be taken at a particular time of day? For how long do I need to take it and why?

_____

_____

_____

Do I call the doctor or go to the emergency room if I feel sick or think I have a reaction to any medications?

_____

_____

_____

Are there any programs I can enroll in to help me lose weight, stop smoking, reduce stress, or learn to prepare food in a healthier way?

_____

_____

_____

Whom in the office should I call if I have additional questions?

_____

_____

_____

Remember, you should always follow your doctor's instructions and take your medication as prescribed. Don't try to second-guess your treatment. If you have questions or you think different aspects of your healthcare are causing you to have problems, tell your doctor. Only you know how you feel, but it's your physician and the other professionals in your physician's office who can help you solve any problems.

YOUR HEALTHCARE TEAM: WHO'S WHO?

There was a time when the only people on your healthcare team were the doctor, the receptionist, and a nurse to take your blood pressure and pulse. Times have changed. The modern medical office employs a number of people with various degrees and qualifications. So how do you know who's who? The following is a comprehensive list of the people you may find tending to your health needs, depending on the size of the practice.

The physician (MD or DO) is the person in the office with the most training and is the one in charge. Doctors have anywhere from three to seven years of training after medical school.

The nurse practitioner / clinical nurse specialist (NP/CNS) is a registered nurse with a master's or doctoral degree and five hundred to seven hundred hours of direct patient care. The NP/CNS has acquired the knowledge and clinical competence to diagnose medical problems, prescribe medications, order treatments, and perform advanced medical procedures. Depending on the state in which he or she is licensed, an NP/CNS may or may not work independently of a physician. The training of an NP/CNS strongly emphasizes disease prevention and health management.

The physician assistant (PA) is licensed to practice medicine as part of a team supervised by a physician. PAs can prescribe medication in some states, order treatments and lab tests, and diagnose illnesses and injuries. Most have a master's degree in addition to two thousand hours of training with patients as part of their schooling.

The registered nurse (RN) is licensed by the state. Although RNs administer medication, care for patients, and administer some procedures, they do so under the direction and guidance of a physician.

Medical students spend time rotating through doctors' offices as part of their training, so you may not see the same one twice. These students interact with patients by taking medical histories and may assist the doctor, but they cannot prescribe medication or perform tests on their own.

The technician ("tech") is a medical professional who holds an associate's degree in clinical laboratory science and is qualified to draw blood and perform routine medical tests, such as EKGs and mammograms. The tests techs perform are dictated by the specialty of the medical practice in which they work. Techs work under the supervision of a doctor.

DON'T FORGET THE DENTIST

Another important doctor in your life is your dentist. You may not associate regular dental appointments with heart health, but people who suffer from periodontal (gum) disease are almost twice as likely to suffer from coronary artery disease. The science points to the fact that bacteria in the mouth affects the heart by entering the bloodstream and attaching to fatty plaques in the heart's blood vessels, which contributes to clot formation. As you have learned, blood clots can obstruct normal blood flow and restrict the nutrients and oxygen required for the heart to function properly, which can lead to a heart attack. Another possibility is that the inflammation caused by periodontal disease increases plaque buildup (this is different from the plaque that forms on your teeth), which may contribute to the swelling of the arteries.

Periodontal disease can also worsen existing heart conditions. If you suffer from a heart condition, be sure to inform your dentist. If you are seeing a cardiologist, make sure to let them know when you are going to see the dentist because you will need to be evaluated to determine if your heart condition requires that you take antibiotics prior to your dental procedures (including cleanings).

It's important to practice good oral hygiene: brush twice a day and floss every night. Don't forget to get your teeth cleaned at least once a year, but every six months is better.

Make a plan to identify the professionals who will support your goal of leading a heart-healthy life. Schedule appointments and prepare the questions you'll want to ask. Build partnerships with your doctor, dentist, and the other medical professionals in your life. They are there to help you.

The Importance of Friends and Family

This week, we've focused on building partnerships with your health-care team, but nothing can substitute for the love and support you'll get from your friends and family. These are the partnerships that are vital for well-being, for connection and engagement in the world. But what you might not know is how important these individuals are when it comes to maintaining your health.

Women who seek out the help and support of their friends and family stay motivated and are more successful in achieving their goals. The more people you reach out to in your circle—family, friends, neighbors, church members—the more successful you will be at meeting your goals of leading a healthier life. You won't always have someone around to reward you with praise every time you make a healthy food choice, cook instead of stopping for fast food, or exercise instead of lounging around the house, but if your friends and family members are aware of what you're doing, they are likely to notice, encourage, and compliment you on the positive changes.

Maybe you are lucky enough to have people within your circle who will follow your example and join you for regular walks or adopt the rules for healthy cooking (especially at holidays and family gatherings). As you reach out, you'll find ways to share what you've learned with others, who will likely be very interested once they see the results in the form of a healthier, more fit you.

Begin by choosing the kind of support that you need—the kind that will help you achieve your goals. Next, think about the right person who can provide it—someone who can give you positive reinforcement or even join you. Don't be shy about enlisting different people for different behaviors. Your sister might not be the best influence when it comes to refusing dessert, but a friend or workmate might. Perhaps a neighbor instead of your spouse will be the one to join you for an evening walk, and you might even motivate each other.

This week, your focus has been on building a support team—the partnerships that will ensure that you can reach your heart-healthy goals. Now, take time to log your achievements in your journal or notebook. Set a goal to schedule a well-woman visit or a dental checkup. Find a buddy and schedule a walk. Remember to look back and review your entries every week so you have proof of just how much you've progressed. When you reach a milestone—a good blood pressure reading, stable blood sugar numbers, lower cholesterol level, or even dropping a pound or two—reward yourself. You deserve it. Nothing motivates like success!

Week 5

S: SLEEP MORE, STRESS LESS, AND SAVOR LIFE

Getting enough sleep is essential for a healthy heart. Too little sleep disturbs the body's chemistry and can cause you to be tired, irritable, depressed, and susceptible to weight gain, all of which can lead to health issues. For example, the hormone that regulates hunger is suppressed when we're tired, resulting in inactivity and overeating. Both of these things can lead to weight gain and other risks for heart disease, such as hypertension and diabetes.

We all need to get sufficient sleep *every night*. We know you're busy—you have family to take care of, problems on the job, housework—but if you deprive yourself of sleep, you will shorten your life, and that is no exaggeration.

It doesn't matter if the reason you're not getting enough sleep is because you stay up too late or because you are unable to get to sleep or stay asleep. The end result is the same, and it is detrimental to your emotional and physical well-being.

In addition, if you suffer from depression, diabetes, high blood pressure, high cholesterol, or other problems brought about by lack of sleep, those problems and the medications used to treat them can also lead to difficulty sleeping. So it is vital it to make getting enough sleep a priority before you get caught up in an unhealthy cycle. If you are already experiencing these problems sleeping, our Six S.T.E.P.S. Program can help you overcome them.

Adequate Sleep = Heart Health

Consistently getting a good night's sleep is good for the brain and the heart. Sleep recharges, repairs, and rejuvenates the body. Adequate sleep keeps the entire body functioning efficiently and looking good (yes, "beauty sleep" is real).

In a 2020 study published in the journal *Circulation*, researchers found that sleep is an important marker of cardiovascular health.[17] Their results confirmed that poor-quality sleep puts individuals at significantly higher risk of developing high blood pressure, which—as you've learned—is a risk factor for heart disease.

CONSISTENTLY GETTING A GOOD NIGHT'S SLEEP IS GOOD FOR THE BRAIN AND THE HEART.

So, how much is enough? The American Heart Association says that most people need seven hours of sleep a night.[18]

---

17   Nour Makarem et al., "The Role of Sleep as a Cardiovascular Health Metric," *Circulation* March 2, 2020, https://www.ahajournals.org/doi/10.1161/circ.141.suppl_1.36.

18   "Sleep, Women and Heart Disease," American Heart Association, accessed November 16, 2021, https://www.heart.org/en/healthy-living/go-red-get-fit/sleep-women-and-heart-disease.

Less than six hours of sleep a night is particularly harmful, leading to higher blood levels of stress hormones and substances that indicate inflammation, factors that can substantially increase your risk of developing heart disease.[19]

Insufficient sleep makes us prone to accidents, bad moods, and depression and less able to deal with stressful situations, all have which has been shown to increase risk for heart problems. It's ironic that when we're not feeling well, are stressed out, or are pressed for time, we tend to get less sleep, even though that is when we actually need it the most. This chapter will help you understand and overcome common sleep issues. If you can't fall asleep or stay asleep, make this a top priority to discuss with your doctor. Your health truly depends on it.

Not getting enough sleep:

- Interferes with glucose metabolism leading to insulin resistance, which raises the risk of type 2 diabetes

- Affects production of growth hormones and stress hormones

- Increases risk of high blood pressure

- Makes it difficult to control emotions and stress

- Leads to inability to concentrate and make competent decisions

- Influences the production of the hormone that regulates hunger

- Reduces physical activity, which reduces energy expenditure and leads to weight gain

---

19   "A good night's sleep: Advice to take to heart," Harvard Health Publishing, September 1, 2017, https://www.health.harvard.edu/heart-health/a-good-nights-sleep-advice-to-take-to-heart.

- Increases LDL (bad) cholesterol and lowers HDL (good) cholesterol

- Interferes with metabolizing of some medications

The good news is that with some lifestyle changes you can get enough sleep and wake refreshed every morning. Read on!

How to Get That Full Night's Sleep

Developing good sleep habits is the best way to get a full night's sleep. Many people who complain of not being able to sleep don't really have a medical condition; they just need to modify the everyday behaviors that sabotage their ability to get restful sleep. The following lifestyle changes can make getting a full night's sleep a reality:

- Avoid stimulants like caffeine or nicotine within three hours of going to bed. Also know that caffeine consumed at any time of day can disrupt a night's sleep. Caffeine is found in soft drinks, iced tea, and even chocolate, so rethink eating that evening chocolate bar or drinking that cup of hot chocolate before bed.

- Avoid alcohol within three hours of going to bed. Although alcohol may allow you to fall asleep more quickly, it reduces REM (rapid eye movement) sleep. REM happens about ninety minutes after we fall asleep and is thought to be restorative. Disruptions in REM sleep may cause daytime drowsiness and poor concentration.

- Don't nap for more than twenty to thirty minutes (and not too late in the day).

- Soak up some rays. Daylight promotes melatonin production, which regulates sleep and mood. Either get outdoors every morning or afternoon or get a full-spectrum light (to simulate sunlight) for your home or office.

- Stay active. Make sure to move around during the day and expend enough energy to tire yourself out so you're able to sleep at bedtime.

- Set regular wake and bedtimes. Try to go to bed at the same time every night and get up at the same time every morning—even on weekends.

- Turn off your mind. Take time to unwind or practice a relaxing bedtime ritual that functions to separate waking time from sleeping time. Try reading a book, listening to soft music, or just spending some quiet time alone, away from noise and bright lights and electronic devices.

- Put away electronic visual devices. Switch off computers, tablets, and smartphones at least an hour before bedtime, because the light they emit activates the mind, which will keep you awake.

- Don't drink liquids too close to bedtime, as this can make you get up during the night to use the bathroom.

- Check your medications. Some high blood pressure medications, steroids, antidepressants, decongestants, and other drugs can interfere with the quality of or ability to sleep. Discuss these issues with your doctor to see if the dosage timing can be changed or if an appropriate substitute can be prescribed.

- Regulate bedroom temperature, lighting, and noise level. It's best to sleep in a cool, dark, quiet room. Use eyeshades, blackout curtains, and/or foam earplugs if needed.

- Eat at least two hours before you go to bed and if, for medical reasons, you must eat something close to bedtime, make it light.

- Use your bed for sleeping and sex—*only*. Your bed is not the place to do work, homework, or anything else that does not involve pleasure, rest, or relaxation, ultimately ending in sleep.

- Replace an old mattress or pillow to make your bed more inviting and comfortable. You'll look forward to going to bed when it provides a luxurious end to a long day.

HELLO, SLEEP!

If you find yourself struggling to fall asleep—or if you toss and turn throughout the night—it may be time to examine your bedtime habits and establish some new routines. Your phone can be an obstacle or a valuable ally in sleeping longer and better. Here are three simple tech tweaks that you can try to see how they impact your sleep:

- **Consider the night shift.** Your screen's blue light is easy on the eyes—unless you're trying to fall asleep. Then, that steady stream of light acts just like sunshine streaming through a window, convincing you that it's not bedtime. Place it somewhere out of reach so that you're not tempted to pick it up "just to check." If you must keep it near your bed, dim that light. Most smartphones have a "night shift" option—check display and brightness in your settings. You can use that to schedule a time when your phone's display will shift to warmer colors every evening.

- **Set your alarm.** Use your phone's alarm not simply to wake you up but also to remind you to go to bed. Test out your phone's Health app to set a regular sleep schedule—and when your phone signals that it's time for sleep, pay attention!

- **Schedule downtime.** If you have good intentions to limit your screen time before bed but find it difficult to resist the temptation of a few more minutes on Instagram or checking email, use your phone to schedule time away from the screen. Go to Screen Time in your settings; you can schedule a specific downtime, set time limits on your apps, or pause messages and phone calls while you are sleeping.

Keep a Sleep Journal

Keeping a sleep journal may help you to identify what is causing or contributing to your sleep issues:

- Keep track of medications, activities, and events in your life to see what is causing the problem.

- Use a section in your notebook as a sleep journal. Record the time you go to bed and the time you wake up. Note if you fell asleep right away or not, if and when you woke up during the night, and why and the total number of hours you were actually asleep.

- Note how you feel each morning when you wake up (refreshed, tired, feeling foggy, etc.) and note anything that kept you awake or disrupted your sleep, including troubling thoughts of work, family, or friends; a disturbing dream or pain; trouble breathing; a restless pet; light from another room or a street lamp; noisy neighbors/family; etc.

- Make a note before bed of how much caffeine, alcohol, or medications you took, what time you ate dinner, how long and what time of day you exercised, and how long you were outdoors.

- Note if you felt sleepy during the day. If you took a nap, note the time and for how long.

- Record your nightly bedtime routine (taking a shower, reading a book, meditating, checking your phone or email, etc.).

- Keep the log for at least a week, but longer is better, to help isolate what is interfering with your ability to have a good night's sleep.

- Share your sleep log with your doctor if your journal doesn't provide you with the answers you need and you are still at a loss as to why you cannot sleep.

Also use your journal to identify things that cause you stress and then follow the relaxation techniques we outline later in this chapter. Once you find a technique that works, practice it every day. It will give you the chance to unwind and get on with your day. Finally, if you cannot overcome sleeplessness or anxiety/stress or are kept awake by an active mind, nightmares, sleepwalking, snoring, inability to breathe, pain, or other physical problems, make it a priority to talk to your doctor.

Helpful Hints for Restless Nights

If you're one of the fortunate ones who doesn't often have trouble sleeping but has the occasional restless night (perhaps when there is something important happening the next day), try this. Get out of bed and out of the bedroom and do something relaxing and nonstimulating that will free your mind. Read a book, listen to soft music, or pet your cat until you feel tired enough to go back to bed.

When You Need Help Getting to Sleep

This goes for everyone: resist the urge to take an over-the-counter sleep aid and **never** "borrow" prescription medication from a friend or family member. Not only do you run the risk of a sleep medication interfering with medications you are already taking, but some can leave you feeling foggy the next day, which is the opposite of what you want or need. If you and your physician ultimately determine that you will benefit from taking a sleep medication, follow your doctor's instructions and use only as prescribed.

Seven? Eight? How Many Hours Is Enough?

Earlier, we noted the American Heart Association's recommendation of seven hours a day of sleep. You may have heard that eight hours was the magic number, but in reality it varies from person to person. The average adult needs at least seven hours, but many women do best with eight hours or more—especially when recovering from an illness. The key to knowing if you've had enough sleep is if you wake refreshed each morning and ready to start your day.

Getting an adequate amount of rest also provides you with the foundation for being able to problem-solve. Tackling problems head on means they get resolved and go away rather than sticking around and wearing you down. Problems that aren't resolved can create a vicious cycle of stress / sleeplessness / health problems that you cannot afford.

When you awake refreshed, you think clearly and won't be easily overwhelmed. You will stay in a better mood and are more likely to make clearer and stronger choices like maintaining a healthy diet and moving more.

The Power of Napping

Taking a nap can save the day! It doesn't matter whether it's a daily nap or an emergency nap—the rule is that even though a nap can rejuvenate you when you're feeling tired, it's not to be used as a substitute for a good night's sleep. If you nap because you can't sleep through the night, then you have a problem that might require professional help. However, when you need a nap, take a nap. It can be a lifesaver for the occasional sleepless night, when you know you are anticipating a late-night event, or just because you feel like taking a nap on a lazy day.

A nap of twenty to thirty minutes is best for improving alertness and not waking with that groggy feeling. Make sure that you nap early in the afternoon so as not to interfere with your regular bedtime.

Stress Less and Savor Life More

Stress! Stress is a fact of modern life, and there's no way to avoid it completely. But before we denigrate stress altogether, let's remember that some types of stress are actually beneficial because they make us put pressure on ourselves to complete tasks and accomplish what we need to.

UNDERSTANDING STRESS

Stress comes from our body's activation of the "fight-or-flight" mode, which is our instinctive response to dealing with situations we find fearful. This response has helped us to survive through the ages. When the body is in fight-or-flight mode, it secretes adrenaline and cortisol (stress hormone), which cause us to become hyperaware and focused and ready to respond physically and mentally to whatever is coming our way. So stress in its purest form is not a bad thing. However, problems arise when the stress we experience crosses the line from helping us get through the day to preventing us from living a happy and productive life.

Stress, if not controlled, can lead to depression and anxiety and set the stage for unhealthy behaviors that lead to poor health. Over-eating, excessive drinking, and smoking lead to physical issues such as weight gain, diabetes, and high blood pressure—all the major risk factors of heart disease. And this is just the tip of the iceberg! Stress can cause irritability, inability to sleep, loss of sense of humor, excessive worrying, physical aches and pains, forgetfulness, depression, and other psychological problems. These are some of the most common, but we are sure you'll be able to name others.

What this means to your overall health is that just as you must control what you eat and how much exercise you get, it's equally important to manage stress and keep it at a healthy level. Although there was some debate in the past on the correlation between stress and heart disease, the American Heart Association has recently published a scientific statement on the importance of mental health to overall health and to heart disease prevention and treatment.

THREE TYPES OF STRESS

Here's how, on a very basic level, stress can lead to heart disease. High levels of stress cause the release of cortisol, causing the heart to beat faster, blood pressure to rise, and blood sugar levels to increase. Elevated levels of cortisol lead to an accumulation of belly fat, increased appetite and a craving for unhealthy, high-calorie foods. Stress is also a factor in causing weight gain because people who are under stress tend to be sedentary. In addition, some people turn to smoking or excessive drinking in an effort to feel better, and both are detrimental to your heart health.

According to the American Psychological Association, there are three different types of stress, each with its own characteristics and symptoms:

- **Acute stress.** This type of stress comes from the demands and pressures of everyday life—for example, the fender bender in the parking lot, the deadline you are rushing to meet, or the coffee that you spilled on your blouse before an important presentation—small, everyday crises that we tend to confront, deal with, and move past. Common symptoms of acute stress are irritability, muscular pain, stomach problems, rapid heart rate, sweaty palms, and heart palpitations.

- **Episodic acute stress.** This type of stress occurs in those who suffer acute stress on a consistent basis, often individuals who are described as type A personalities, or chronic worriers. Common symptoms of episodic acute stress are persistent headaches, chronic high blood pressure, and erratic sleep patterns.

- **Chronic stress.** This type of stress comes from the major problems involved with such issues as taking care of an ailing family member or dealing with your own health issues, not having a job or enough money, and so on. Chronic stress doesn't go away at the end of the day.

HOW STRESS AFFECTS THE HEART

Stress affects the heart by:

- Increasing the heart rate and causing the arteries to constrict, which decreases blood flow

- Increasing certain factors in the blood that can damage the arteries that supply blood and nutrients to the heart

- Making blood sticky and increasing the likelihood of forming an artery-clogging clot, which can lead to a heart attack

- Temporarily raising cholesterol levels, preventing the body from ridding itself of fat molecules

- Influencing cravings for salt, fat, and sugar, which cause weight gain, to counteract tension

- Raising the amount of the hormone cortisol, which is responsible for the accumulation of belly fat

- Worsening diabetes, because insulin, which regulates blood glucose levels, is not able to function appropriately, which causes blood sugar level to rise. Cortisol also increases blood sugar levels.

STRESS IS CAUSED BY "STRESSORS"

Anything that causes stress is called a stressor. Stressors can be minor hassles, minor or major lifestyle changes, or a combination of both. Since every one of us has to deal with stress of some type, the key is to figure out if your stressor is serious enough to impact your health. Take a moment and think about your daily activities at home and work. Because any activity has the potential to cause stress, especially activities caused by physical or emotional changes or changes in daily routine, take an inventory of what is going on in your life. Granted, some changes, although they may be stressful, are actually good for you and will eventually become routine. However, the stressors you need to be aware of are the ones that don't let up and tend to wear you down.

List in your notebook *any* stressors that may be affecting your well-being. The list below will help you to identify some, and there may be some you are experiencing that aren't included:

- Daily hassles (commuting, shopping, cooking, housekeeping, etc.)

- Work overload

- Starting a new job

- Losing a job

- Retirement

- Financial worries

- Legal problems

- Change of residence

- Death of a relative or friend

- Ending a romantic relationship
- Disagreements with family, friends, or coworkers

THE WARNING SIGNS OF TOO MUCH STRESS

If any of the stressors in your life cause any of the following problems, this is an indication that you need to slow down and learn how to disarm that stressor and its unhealthy influence. Whatever you do, do not ignore any of the following warning signs because they are the body's way of telling you that it needs a better way to protect itself from a problem in the making or the worsening of an existing medical problem.

Depending on the severity, you may want to consult with your physician.

- *Physical signs:* Dizziness, aches, pains and muscle spasms, grinding or clenching of teeth, headaches, indigestion, muscle tension, sleeplessness, racing heartbeat, ringing in the ears, sweaty palms, chronic tiredness, exhaustion, trembling, excessive weight loss or gain

- *Emotional signs:* Anxiety, crying, anger, depression, feeling of powerlessness, hopelessness or loneliness, mood swings, irritability, negative outlook, nervousness, sadness

- *Cognitive signs:* Inability to concentrate, loss of sense of humor or inability to laugh, forgetfulness or poor memory, constant worrying, difficulty making decisions, lack of creativity

- *Behavioral signs:* Overeating, compulsive eating, other eating disorders, excessive drinking, smoking or drug use, quick temper, impulsive actions, constantly criticizing others, frequent job changes, withdrawal from personal relationships or social situations

HOW TO DIAL DOWN THE STRESS

We have provided you with a lot of information regarding stress and its effects on your health. Once you identify your stressors, you can better manage them, thereby lessening their toll on your health. On the following page are twelve ways to reduce stress; you should choose the ones that work for you. Like anything else, there is more than one fix for everyone or every problem, and trial and error will show you which works best. If you are experiencing chronic stress due to unemployment, illness, or family dysfunction, these techniques may help with some of your symptoms, but more focused medical and behavioral treatment may also be indicated. Nevertheless, these techniques can still help you relax and calm your mind, thereby lessening the impact of stress on your health. Again, make sure you let your physician know if the stress is overwhelming and basic stress reduction techniques are not sufficiently helpful.

> ONCE YOU IDENTIFY YOUR STRESSORS, YOU CAN BETTER MANAGE THEM, THEREBY LESSENING THEIR TOLL ON YOUR HEALTH.

1. **Reach out and enjoy time with friends and family.** You don't have to go it alone! Develop a supportive circle of trusting people and you'll always have someone there to listen when you need to talk about what's bothering you or you want to share some good news. If you're feeling lonely, call someone—sometimes you have to make the first move.

2. **Breathe deeply.** Learning how to breathe deeply instead of shallowly from your chest (the routine way) is an important step in managing stress. With deep breathing, you really fill up your lungs with air and then let it out slowly in a smooth, even, rhythmic way. This type of deep diaphragm breathing

promotes a good exchange of oxygen coming into the lungs with the waste product, carbon dioxide, going out. It helps the body to relax by stopping the fight-or-flight response and also has the ability to release its own built-in painkillers. You may wish to try the breathing exercise we've provided in the box.

TAKE A BREATH

One of the simplest steps you can take to manage stress more effectively is through the practice of focused deep breathing.

Try this easy exercise from Harvard Medical School to help you focus on your breath while setting aside stressful thoughts and feelings:[20]

- Find a quiet place where you can comfortably sit or lie down.

- First, take a normal breath.

- Next, focus on taking a deep breath, breathing in slowly through your nose. Pay attention to the sensation of your chest and lower belly rising as you inhale.

- Breathe out slowly through your mouth or nose, whichever feels more natural.

- Try a pattern of five deep breaths, inhaling for a count of five and exhaling for a count of five.

---

20 "Relaxation techniques: Breath control helps quell errant stress response," Harvard Health Publishing, July 6, 2020, https://www.health.harvard.edu/mind-and-mood/relaxation-techniques-breath-control-helps-quell-errant-stress-response.

If you wish, as you sit or lie comfortably with your eyes closed, combine this deep breathing with helpful imagery, fixing in your mind a picture or place where you feel relaxed and at peace.

3. **Stop feeling rushed.** Make sure you allow yourself the time you need to get to where you are going and to do what you need to do. By allowing yourself five to ten minutes more time than you think you need to perform any task, you can take the pressure off yourself. It's amazing the difference this one small change can make in improving the quality of your life.

4. **Schedule wisely and make lists.** Take a look at your calendar, and if there's no white space in it, build in rest stops between appointments, chores, and trips. That includes weekends and holidays. Keep a running and up-to-date to-do list so nothing will take you by surprise.

5. **Stick to your schedule.** Nothing can make you more stressed than the demands on your time by others. You've made a schedule; now stick to it by learning to say no. Of course you need to be realistic and flexible, and there will be exceptions, but they should be just that—exceptions. Be creative with your time, figure out shortcuts, and don't procrastinate. Do the big jobs when you're fresh and the less important things when you're tired and don't have much brainpower left. When you're organized, you'll have more time to do the things that energize and destress.

6. **Declutter and organize your living and work spaces.**
Trying to live and function in a cluttered and disorganized house or office can drain your energy and cause you additional stress. Think about the anxiety you feel when you can't find something in a hurry (or at all). The stress this causes is as real as the precious time it wastes. Declutter your life so it's easy to find what you need.

7. **Get moving / stretch.** Take a walk, stretch in the shower (hot water loosens the muscles), or move around in any way you can. A good stretch or exercise session releases stored tension and makes you feel more relaxed and energized, ready to handle whatever comes your way.

8. **Schedule time to do what gives you joy.** Perhaps it's reading, gardening, seeing friends, taking a bath, going for a walk, watching TV, or spending quiet time with a pet. Pare down your to-do list and carve out some time to go out to dinner, to a movie, or out with the girls. The point is to take a break from your regular routine, so block out this time as the important appointment it is. If you have set aside time to knit every Thursday at noon, then on Wednesday evening be certain to have your yarn, pattern, and the correct-size needles ready and waiting. Think of it as your "prescription" for health. Look through your calendar; we're sure you'll find some time for yourself!

9. **Prioritize and delegate.** There are always tasks and chores that you can ask family, friends, or coworkers to help you do. Of course there are things that you must do yourself, but the point is that you don't need to do it all, all the time. Understanding this will alleviate stress and guilt. For example, if

you walk your child to school, maybe you can share this responsibility with another parent or parents. Chances are that they will welcome the free time it brings them too. Learn to ask for help when you need it. You can also make your life simpler by taking some of those chores off your current to-do list. Just as you don't need to do everything yourself, you don't need to do everything at once.

10. **Learn when "good enough" is good enough.** Sometimes we need to learn to settle for a result that is acceptable rather than always pursuing perfection. For example, getting the family together for dinner is more important than serving the perfect meal. If that means stopping at the local delicatessen to pick up a salad rather than making a home-cooked meal, consider that good enough!

11. **Get enough sleep.** You won't be able to cope with the trials of daily living or, in fact, any particularly stressful situations if you're not well rested.

12. **Practice relaxation techniques including meditation, biofeedback, and visualization.** These relaxation techniques have been proven to reduce anxiety and the severity of congestive heart failure and headaches as well as control blood pressure, and they may even help prevent heart attacks and strokes and lower adrenaline levels, which also helps the heart. There are many reputable websites that can help you learn these techniques, such as www.nimh.nih.gov, www.heart.org, and www.mayoclinic.org.

MINDFUL MEDITATION

Dr. Herbert Benson, cardiologist and founder of Harvard's Mind/Body Medical Institute, is among the many researchers who promote meditation as a way to reduce stress and improve heart health. Dr. Benson describes the practice of focused breathing and meditation as a way to inspire what he calls "the relaxation response."[21]

Try this simple meditation practice as a way to begin:

- Sit quietly with your eyes closed and focus on your breathing, inhaling deeply and then slowly exhaling.

- If you find it helpful, focus on the word "peace" and repeat it silently to yourself each time you exhale.

- Whenever you become aware of a stray thought distracting you, quietly promise to return to that thought later, and then repeat the word "peace."

This exercise will help you begin to practice an awareness of the present and an ability to set aside stressful thoughts and distractions. Start by spending a few minutes each day, and gradually extend the time you dedicate to mindful relaxation.

SOME STRESS-BUSTING ACTIVITIES

Sometimes we need to take time out from our already full, stressed-out lives and do something fun to relieve stress. When we feel happy, it's easier to tackle life's daily challenges. Women tend to put their

---

21   "The magic of mindfulness," Harvard Health Publishing, September 1, 2013, https://www.health.harvard.edu/staying-healthy/the-magic-of-mindfulness.

own needs last, and consequently, things that make them happy can fall by the wayside. It's like being on a hamster wheel. Once it's going around, it's hard to get off, but you must stop the wheel and set aside time for yourself. Here are some examples:

- **Get a hobby.** We're sure you have things you've always wanted to do, learn, or try, and now that you've scheduled the time, do it! Drawing or painting, cards and games, knitting, needle-point, crocheting, crosswords, and sudoku are all great stress relievers. Gardening is also a great hobby, and it gets you outdoors. Remember, a hobby is *any activity* done in your leisure time that gives you enjoyment. That's its sole purpose!

- **Schedule "me" time.** Maybe you don't want a hobby; maybe what you need is time for yourself to do nothing in particular. That's great; just make sure you do it. Take a long bath, call a friend on the phone, or meet someone for breakfast, lunch, or dinner. Go to a movie alone, take a walk, or read a book. Just make sure that it's something you enjoy, that it's a break from your regular routine, and that doing it will make you feel good.

- **Listen to (or play) music.** Listening to music reduces stress and improves mental and physical health. What's great about this activity is that you can do it any time, even while you're doing other things. Turn on the radio, listen to your iPhone, or put on your favorite playlist and absorb the positive energy that comes from listening to music. Music also complements other healthy lifestyle habits by adding a sense of peace, putting a spring into your step, or stimulating your mind, so take your music on your morning walk or have it on in the background as you read or write in your journal or exercise or cook dinner. If you play an instrument, that's the perfect way to let the music work its magic.

- **Take time to laugh.** Laughter is good for your health. We're not kidding. Read some jokes on the internet, call a friend, learn a joke, watch a funny movie, whatever it takes. Laughing actually causes healthy changes in the body. It relaxes the body, decreases production of stress hormones, produces antibodies to help boost the immune system, triggers the production of endorphins that reduce pain, and protects against heart attack by improving blood flow. Laughing also helps us to bond with others. Follow our prescription and take advantage of this free medicine—at least once a day!

- **Reward yourself.** We are talking about treating yourself to something special that doesn't necessarily cost money. For example, light some candles and take a long bath, have a pajama night on the couch watching that movie you've been meaning to see, or schedule a stop at your library to stock up on the latest fun reads.

MAINTAIN A POSITIVE ATTITUDE AND SELF-ESTEEM

More than anything, maintaining a positive attitude and good self-esteem gives you the wherewithal to view stress as a *challenge* rather than a *problem*. A positive attitude helps you when you encounter situations beyond your control, because it gives you the courage to accept and make the best of those situations. The following will help you better manage life's stress:

- **Stay calm.** Stop before you react. Breathe deeply. Rationally evaluate the choices available to you.

- **Give yourself a pep talk.** You can get through this situation.

- **Keep everything in perspective.** Consider possible solutions and act on one that is acceptable and feasible.

- **Prepare for the worst but hope for the best.** Never give up hope. Odds are that things will not be as bad as you imagine.

- **Appreciate the experience.** There is always a lesson to be learned. Anything you can learn, even from a difficult situation, can help you in the future.

- **Start each day with a healthy breakfast.** A well-balanced meal of protein, whole grains, or complex carbs and fruit maintains blood sugar levels to give you the sustenance and strength to think clearly. If you need to eat on the run, instant oatmeal (no sugar added!), granola, fruit, and low-fat yogurt are good choices.

- **Take life one day at a time.** No matter how bad things seem, every day is a new day. Stress won't disappear from your life, but a positive attitude will help you manage it and prepare for what comes your way.

As you complete Week 5, it's important to recognize and appreciate the healthy changes you are making. Congratulations on your progress. Keep up the good work.

TAKE CARE OF YOURSELF

This week, make a conscious choice to spend time practicing new habits that will help you reduce stress and begin to savor your life more. Use this worksheet to identify the self-care practices that work for you, and note the results as a way to inspire yourself to keep up the good work!

This week I did the following:

☐ Put away all screens and devices an hour before going to sleep

☐ Set a bedtime reminder

☐ Took a twenty-minute nap

☐ Practiced focused breathing

☐ Practiced mindful meditation

☐ Added an hour to my schedule for an activity that gives me joy

☐ Experimented with delegating more tasks

☐ Decluttered my living or work space

☐ Scheduled fun time with family or friends

☐ Said no to an unscheduled request

Add any observations you've made as a result of these practices: _____

_____

_____

_____

_____

You may find wish to add a specific daily or weekly appointment in your calendar to continue the self-care practices that you found especially helpful.

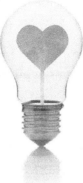

Week 6

PERMANENT S.T.E.P.S. TO
A HEALTHIER HEART

You're finally there! It's time to put into practice the heart-smart lifestyle changes you learned over the past five weeks. Remember those "small steps" mentioned at the beginning of this book? Integrating these new behaviors into your life will make them your new habits, and your new habits will soon become permanent.

Sasha and Chandra

Earlier in this book, we shared the stories of Claudia, the forty-eight-year-old banker, and Rebecca, the thirty-four-year-old nurse. Now, we'd like to spend a few minutes with two other women: Sasha and Chandra.

Let's start first with Sasha. As you may remember, Sasha is a fifty-nine-year-old Black woman who cares for her mother at home.

Recently, she had been experiencing bouts of indigestion and nausea. She initially assumed that she had the flu, but when her symptoms continued, she wisely contacted her doctor, who, after tests and screening, informed her that her symptoms are actually warning signs of a blockage in her coronary artery. Thankfully, Sasha and her doctors caught this in time and were able to address the problem by performing an emergency procedure in which they implanted a stent in Sasha's artery. However, the stent procedure is not where Sasha's journey to a healthier heart ends, but rather where it begins.

Chandra is a thirty-three-year-old woman of South Asian descent whose work as an assistant to a department store president extends well beyond a typical nine-to-five day. Her commute to work is long, and she frequently skips breakfast in order to arrive on time. She knows that she should focus more on healthy eating habits, but she is surprised when, during an annual gynecological appointment, her doctor notes that she has high blood pressure and explains that having both high blood pressure and diabetes places her at an increased risk for cardiovascular disease.

Sasha and Chandra both decided to follow the Six S.T.E.P.S. Program, recognizing the importance of choosing to develop heart-healthy habits for lifetime wellness. Chandra learned that despite her busy schedule, her apartment must be stocked with healthy snack choices, whole fruits, vegetables, and healthy fats and that breakfast must be part of her daily meal planning. She engaged the help of her roommate, who located several farmers markets in the area, and they decided to take turns doing the weekly shopping and stocking the kitchen with heart-healthy choices. As she experimented with new, healthy options, she discovered that she enjoyed cooking and found meal preparation a great way to relax at the end of the day.

To ensure that she made time in her schedule for breakfast, Chandra recognized that she needed to focus more on her sleep schedule. A few simple changes made a big difference; she set a sleep alarm on her phone and used it as a reminder to put down her devices and get ready for bed. Gradually, she adjusted to the earlier bedtime and discovered that, with a healthy breakfast, her energy levels were higher throughout the day—and she found the daily commute less stressful.

Sasha also committed to purging her home of processed foods and restocking her refrigerator with healthy foods she and her mother could enjoy. As a caregiver, Sasha had always put the needs of others above her own, but with the encouragement of her doctor, she began to carve out time each day for meditation and exercise. Before joining a gym, she decided to make sure that she took ten thousand steps every day. She purchased an inexpensive step tracker and began measuring all of her daily steps. She realized that there are countless opportunities to add steps to her day without significantly changing her schedule, and she actually enjoyed the feeling of accomplishment and good health she was achieving. She parked her car at the far end of the parking lot when she went to the grocery store; she took a short walk every day after lunch while her mother napped; and she took a second walk in the evening while listening to a podcast. She enjoyed the satisfaction of meeting her goal each day, and the added exercise gave Sasha more energy and helped her sleep more soundly.

Sasha and Chandra are success stories. They have continued to follow our program and to make small but meaningful choices to live healthier lives. Now, it's time for your success story.

On Your Way to Heart Health

Sasha and Chandra's examples demonstrate that it is possible to make simple changes to your life, even if you have a demanding job or are caring for a family member. Although these changes seem small, they are crucial to getting you on the road to health and overall wellness. You can make these changes gradually, but making them is essential if you are going to live a heart-smart life. Once you start seeing the benefits (and you will), it will become increasingly easy to maintain these new habits. These simple small steps will help you to arrive at a healthier lifestyle and become truly heart smart!

Week 6 is the time to review your successes and evaluate where you have opportunities for improvement. It's important to celebrate those successes and be proud of them. But you will also learn a lot from your failures when you identify what didn't work and understand why.

Looking back over the past five weeks, think about your successes and challenges and record them in your notebook. Did you have a harder time with changing your eating habits than with exercise or managing stress? Was it easy for you to choose to eat healthier food? As you moved on to Week 2 and added exercise, perhaps you made great strides with your new exercise routine but had challenges maintaining that healthier eating routine. Don't worry. It is common for one aspect of the program to work better than another when taking on new lifestyle changes over a fairly short period of time. Your commitment to living a heart-smart life is a long-term commitment, and your journal will be a valuable tool to help you get there. We've included a worksheet at the end of this chapter; use it to set new goals, reflect on areas that have been challenging, and celebrate the positive changes you've made during the past six weeks. Remember, small steps will make a big difference, so recognize and take pride in every healthy meal you've eaten, that extra walk you're taking in the evening, and the well-woman visit you've scheduled with your healthcare provider. We are celebrating with you!

WEEK 6 REFLECTIONS

I've noticed the following changes in my overall well-being as a result of the Six S.T.E.P.S. Program: _____

_____

_____

_____

I've noticed these changes in my sleep patterns: _____

_____

_____

_____

I've noticed these changes in my energy levels:_____

_____

_____

_____

This is my favorite new breakfast: _____

_____

_____

_____

I've discovered that I really enjoy this: _____

_____

_____

_____

Moving more is easier when I do this: _____

_____

_____

_____

My most challenging change during the program was my
choice to commit to this: _____

_____

_____

_____

Going forward, I'm inspired to try this: _____

_____

_____

_____

During my Week 7, I'm eager to do this: _____

_____

_____

_____

For the next six weeks, I'm choosing to take steps toward
these goals: _____

_____

_____

_____

I want to celebrate this part of my success story: _____

_____

_____

_____

PART THREE

GET SMARTER—ELEVATE YOUR HEART IQ

"When I dare to be powerful, to use my strength in the service of my vision, then it becomes less and less important whether I am afraid."
—AUDRE LORDE

Congratulations on choosing to make your health a priority and for committing to taking steps each day to care for yourself and your heart!

The Six S.T.E.P.S. Program offers insight and encouragement to support you as you start moving toward a heart-healthy life. But the six weeks are only the beginning. Selecting healthy foods, prioritizing exercise and sleep, partnering with your healthcare provider … these are choices that will create positive change for years to come.

In the pages that follow, you'll find additional resources and information that will be helpful as you move forward. We'll share suggestions to boost your meal planning with a week of heart-healthy menus. You'll have the opportunity to learn more about healthy portion control. You'll find tips for simple exercises you can practice to build strength and flexibility—no gym membership required. Plus you'll discover information that can help you build more knowledge about how to develop a heart-healthy lifestyle.

We said it earlier—supportive partnerships matter. We've built a community of women just like you—women who are taking the steps and celebrating the successes and cheering through the challenges of heart-healthy living. We want you to be a part of that community. You'll find more information at the end of this book and on our website.

Now, let's get started elevating your heart IQ.

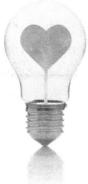

Nourish

A WEEK'S WORTH OF DELICIOUS, EASY MENUS FOR YOUR HEART HEALTH

We understand that it can be challenging to choose heart-healthier meal options. But the good news is that we're not talking about dieting or depriving yourself of delicious foods. There are many heart-healthy options that are nourishing *and* satisfying—foods that you'll look forward to eating and will want to add to your weekly meal planning.

To help you get started, Registered Dietitian Marissa Licata has created this menu as a guideline for a week of heart-healthy eating. Use this as a guide to demonstrate how to balance meals and snacks. Feel free to mix and match different options to suit your budget and taste preferences. Make your own substitutions to adapt this to your family. Most moderately active women need approximately 1,800 calories per day to maintain their current body weight. If you are trying to drop some pounds however, between 1,200 and 1,600 calories is typical for most women to promote weight loss. This can vary based on your frame and activity level. It is important to stay within a daily calorie budget and choose wholesome, quality foods to fill those daily calories. A food diary app can help you achieve this, and we recommend meeting with a registered dietitian to help you determine your specific calorie goals.

Remember to follow the Six S.T.E.P.S. guidelines for heart-healthy cooking techniques. Share recipes and photos of your tastiest heart-healthy meals with your heart smarter partners, and get inspired.

Monday (Meatless Monday, Remember?)

BREAKFAST

Slice of whole grain toast topped with 1 tablespoon natural peanut butter and 1 small sliced banana, 1 cup nonfat milk or unsweetened dairy alternative

MIDMORNING SNACK

Low-fat cheese stick with whole grain crackers

LUNCH

Salad greens (baby spinach) topped with tomatoes, red peppers, sliced carrots, 1/2 cup garbanzo beans, 1/4 cup wheat berries, 2 to 3 avocado slices, and fresh orange slices. Drizzle with 1 tablespoon extra-virgin olive oil and red wine vinegar, or a squeeze of lemon juice.

DINNER

Roasted halibut (4 ounces) with small baked sweet potato and 1 cup roasted brussels sprouts and 1 cup mixed berries

Tuesday

BREAKFAST

1 cup steel-cut oats topped with 1/2 cup sliced strawberries, 1 table-spoon ground flax seeds or chia seeds, 2 tablespoons crushed walnuts plus 1 hard-boiled egg, and 1 cup nonfat milk or dairy alternative

MIDMORNING SNACK

Medium apple, 1 tablespoon almond butter

LUNCH

2 slices whole-grain bread, 2 slices freshly carved turkey off the bone (note: not lunch meat, which is high in sodium), 1 slice reduced-fat Swiss cheese, topped with lettuce, tomato, and mustard, with carrot sticks on the side, and 1 cup nonfat milk or dairy alternative

DINNER

Grilled shrimp, chicken, or tofu (4 ounces), broccoli, shredded carrots, peas over cauliflower rice

Wednesday

BREAKFAST

2 eggs scrambled with tomatoes, spinach, and onions and 1 slice of toasted whole-grain bread, 1 cup nonfat milk or unsweetened dairy alternative, 1 cup melon balls

MIDMORNING SNACK

3 tablespoons hummus and 1 cup veggie slices (baby carrots, celery, cherry tomatoes, or try something new like jicama slices)

LUNCH

Low-sodium organic or homemade lentil soup, 1 small whole-grain roll, 1 cup red grapes

DINNER

4-ounce grilled salmon with mustard glaze, quinoa, and asparagus (make extra for tomorrow's lunch)

Thursday

BREAKFAST

2 slices whole-grain sprouted bread with 1/2 small smashed avocado and tomato slices, 1 cup of nonfat milk or nondairy alternative

MIDMORNING SNACK

1/2 cup roasted and spiced chickpeas (simply roast them in the oven with your favorite spices) and 1 medium plum

LUNCH

Baby kale topped with grilled salmon (leftover from Wednesday dinner), sliced red pepper, red onions, and radicchio, steamed broccoli florets, with a fresh-squeezed lemon zest/juice and 1 tablespoon extra-virgin olive oil on top, 3 to 4 fresh figs

AFTERNOON SNACK

Whole-grain rice cake with 1 tablespoon almond butter, pear slices, and a sprinkle of chia seeds

DINNER

1 cup chickpea or lentil pasta or 2 cups spaghetti squash topped with homemade ground turkey breast and mushroom marinara sauce

Friday

BREAKFAST

1 cup whole-grain high-fiber cereal topped with nonfat milk or unsweetened dairy alternative and 1/2 cup fresh blueberries

LUNCH

Quinoa bowl topped with fresh corn, red onion, avocado, scallions, cilantro, black beans, squeeze of lime, and 1 tablespoon extra-virgin olive oil, 1/2 cup fresh pineapple

AFTERNOON SNACK

4 ounces nonfat plain yogurt with 1/2 cup fresh raspberries and 1 tablespoon unsalted sunflower seeds

DINNER

Chicken burger in a lettuce wrap (no bun), with farro and tomato salad and roasted string beans. Dessert for a movie night: 3 cups air-popped popcorn with cinnamon or parmesan cheese sprinkle

Saturday

BREAKFAST

Whole-grain toast topped with 1/2 cup part-skim ricotta cheese, fresh cut-up figs, a drizzle of honey (1 teaspoon), and slivered almonds

LUNCH

Homemade pizza: Whole-grain English muffin, rubbed with a garlic clove when warm, 2 slices fresh mozzarella, 2 thick slices of tomato, a drizzle of extra-virgin olive oil, and side salad greens (lettuce, romaine, baby spinach) topped with cucumbers and carrots, drizzle with walnut oil and red wine vinegar

AFTERNOON SNACK

Homemade guacamole with carrot sticks, celery, pepper, and jicama slices

DINNER

Grilled chicken skewers with zucchini, peppers, and onions, chickpea bean salad with red onions, and 1 cup whole wheat couscous. Dessert: Grill 1/2 peach brushed with olive oil and top with 0 percent Greek yogurt and cinnamon, drizzle of 1 tsp honey if desired

Sunday

BREAKFAST

Whole-grain waffle (homemade from 12-grain or 7-grain natural mix) topped with 1 tablespoon natural peanut or almond butter, 1 cup blueberries and raspberries, and 1 teaspoon honey, with 1 cup nonfat milk or dairy alternative

MIDMORNING SNACK

1 cup cantaloupe melon with 1/2 cup low-sodium cottage cheese or reduced-fat Greek yogurt, 1 tablespoon chia seeds

LUNCH

Chicken salad: 4 ounces shredded chicken breast mixed with Dijon mustard, lemon zest, lemon juice, and reduced fat Greek yogurt (replaces mayo), topped with arugula or spinach and tomato in a low-carb, whole-grain wrap and a medium pear

AFTERNOON SNACK

2 mini egg muffin cups with tomato, broccoli, onion, and mushroom

DINNER

Roasted pork tenderloin (4 ounces), with 1/2 cup butternut squash and spinach and radicchio salad with cucumbers, radish, red onion with balsamic vinegar, and 1 tbsp extra-virgin olive oil Dessert: 8 whole strawberries dipped in 2 melted dark chocolate squares

Learn

PORTION SIZE GUIDELINES

If you need extra help interpreting servings and portion sizes, you've come to the right place! On the next few pages, we'll explain how you can measure a healthy serving, and share tips you can use to estimate portions when you're dining out or when a measuring cup isn't handy.

FRUITS AND VEGETABLES

6 to 7 servings per day

1 cup of diced fruit
1 medium-sized whole fruit or vegetable (such as a pear, orange, tomato, or beet)
1/2 cup of cooked or 1 cup raw vegetables
2 cups of raw or 1 cup of cooked leafy green vegetables

BEANS

at least 1 serving per day

1/2 cup cooked beans (can be added to soups or salads or served as a side dish or main course)

GRAINS

5 to 6 servings per day

1/2 cup cooked pasta, brown rice, or other grain or 1 slice of whole-grain bread

PROTEIN

2 ounces at breakfast (such as eggs, cottage cheese, or yogurt) or 4 ounces of lean protein at lunch and dinner

BEVERAGES

8 ounces or more per meal of water, seltzer, herbal tea, tea, or coffee

"Eyeballing" Portion Size

For ease when eating out, there are ways to eyeball the amount of food that constitutes one portion. Commit these basic measurements to memory, or make a copy of these measuring guidelines and post them inside your kitchen cabinet or on the outside the refrigerator door.

THERE ARE WAYS TO EYEBALL THE AMOUNT OF FOOD THAT CONSTITUTES ONE PORTION.

IF MEASURING USING CUPS AND SPOONS:

1 cup = a baseball

1/2 cup = a light bulb

1/4 cup = a large egg

1 ounce or 2 tablespoons = a golf ball

1 tablespoon = half a golf ball

IF COUNTING:

16 grapes = 1/2 cup

23 almonds = 1/4 cup

24 pistachios = 1/4 cup

1 cookie = 1 round tea bag

1 brownie or piece of chocolate = dental floss package

12 baby carrots = 1 cup

8 strawberries = 1 cup

IF MEASURING "BY HAND":

a closed fist = 1 cup / 8 ounces / 227 grams

an open palm (no fingers!) = 2 to 3 ounces / 57 to 85 grams

a whole thumb = 1/8 cup / 2 tablespoons / 1 ounce / 28 grams

a thumb tip = 1 teaspoon / 4 grams

3 thumb tips = 1 tablespoon / 12 grams

WHAT *ONE* SERVING LOOKS LIKE:

3 ounces of lean protein (pork tenderloin, lamb, chicken, tofu) = a deck of cards

3 ounces of fish = a checkbook

1 ounce lunch meat or a pancake = a cell phone

1 white or sweet potato = a deck of cards

1 cup of diced fruit or raw or cooked vegetables = a baseball

1 medium fruit = a baseball

1/2 cup of cooked beans, pasta, rice, or grains = a light bulb

1/2 cup of frozen yogurt, ice cream, or cottage cheese = a light bulb

1 tablespoon of butter, spread, mayo, salad dressing = a K-cup lid

1 1/2 ounces of cheese = 3 stacked dice

2 tablespoons of nuts, dried fruit, hummus, or peanut butter = a golf ball

1 muffin or biscuit = a hockey puck

1 bagel = a small tuna can

1 slice of Italian bread = a deck of cards

3 cups of popcorn = 3 baseballs

Train

STRENGTH AND FLEXIBILITY EXERCISES—NO GYM REQUIRED

To help you kick-start your new fitness routine, here are a few simple strength and flexibility exercises you can try from the comfort of your home, without investing in expensive equipment. Remember to take your time and be patient—you're building new habits and moving your body in new ways!

Before beginning any strength and flexibility routine, you should consult with your physician. Once you are ready to begin your strength and flexibility training, you can use the following information as a general guide to get you started.

Flexibility Exercises

Do each stretching exercise three to five times at each session. Slowly stretch into the desired position, as far as possible without pain, and hold the stretch for ten to thirty seconds. Relax, breathe, then repeat, trying to stretch farther. Here are eight flexibility exercises to get you started:

1. Neck stretch
2. Shoulder and upper arm stretch
3. Upper body stretch
4. Back-of-leg stretch
5. Thigh stretch
6. Hip stretch
7. Lower back stretch
8. Calf stretch

NECK STRETCH

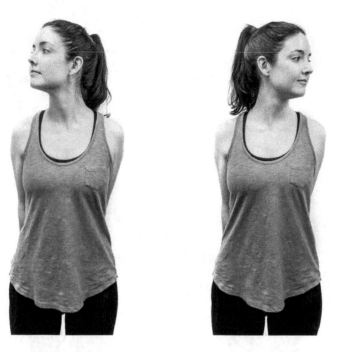

1. Stand or sit in a sturdy chair.

2. Keep your feet flat on the floor, shoulder width apart.

3. Slowly turn your head to the right until you feel a slight stretch. Be careful not to tip or tilt your head forward or backward, but hold it in a comfortable position.

4. Hold the position for ten to thirty seconds.

5. Turn your head to the left and hold the position for ten to thirty seconds.

6. Repeat at least three to five times.

SHOULDER AND UPPER ARM STRETCH

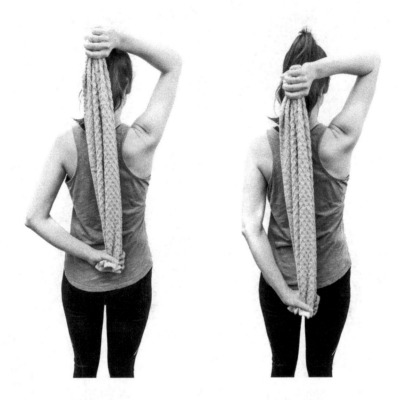

1. Stand with your feet shoulder width apart.

2. Hold one end of a towel in your right hand.

3. Raise and bend your right arm to drape the towel down your back. Keep your right arm in this position and continue holding on to the towel.

4. Reach behind your lower back and grasp the towel with your left hand.

5. To stretch your right shoulder, pull the towel down with your left hand. Stop when you feel a stretch or slight discomfort in your right shoulder.

6. Repeat at least three to five times.

7. Reverse positions and repeat at least three to five times.

UPPER BODY STRETCH

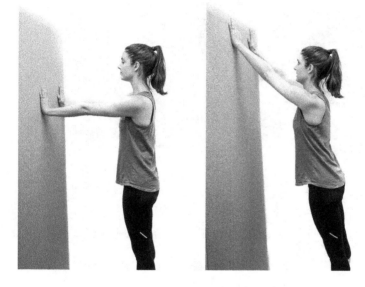

1. Stand facing a wall slightly farther than arm's length away, feet shoulder width apart.

2. Lean your body forward and put your palms flat against the wall at shoulder height and shoulder width apart.

3. Keeping your back straight, slowly walk your hands up the wall until your arms are above your head.

4. Hold your arms overhead for about ten to thirty seconds.

5. Slowly walk your hands back down.

6. Repeat at least three to five times.

BACK-OF-LEG STRETCH

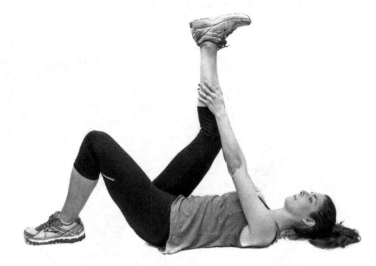

1. Lie on your back with your left knee bent and your left foot flat on the floor.

2. Raise your right leg, keeping your knee slightly bent.

3. Reach up and grasp your right leg with both hands, keeping your head and shoulders flat on the floor.

4. Gently pull your right leg toward your body until you feel a stretch in the back of your leg.

5. Hold position for ten to thirty seconds.

6. Repeat at least three to five times.

7. Repeat at least three to five times with left leg.

THIGH STRETCH

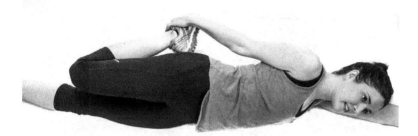

1. Lie on your side with your legs straight and your knees together.

2. Rest your head on your arm.

3. Bend your top knee and reach back and grab the top of your foot. If you can't reach your foot, loop a resistance band, belt, or towel over your foot and hold both ends.

4. Gently pull your leg until you feel a stretch in your thigh.

5. Hold position for ten to thirty seconds.

6. Repeat at least three to five times.

7. Repeat at least three to five times with your other leg.

HIP STRETCH

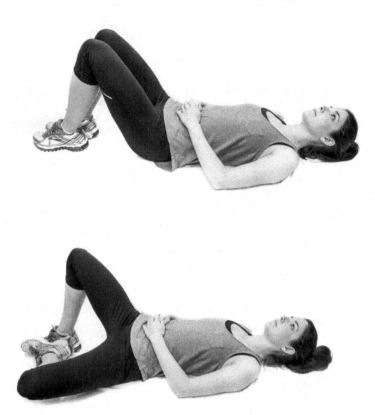

1. Lie on your back with your legs together, knees bent, and
   feet flat on the floor. Try to keep both shoulders on the floor
   throughout the stretch.

2. Slowly lower one knee by opening out to the side as far as
   you comfortably can. Keep your feet close together and try
   not to move the other leg.

3. Hold position for ten to thirty seconds.

4. Bring knee back up slowly.

5. Repeat at least three to five times.

6. Repeat at least three to five times with your other leg.

LOWER BACK STRETCH

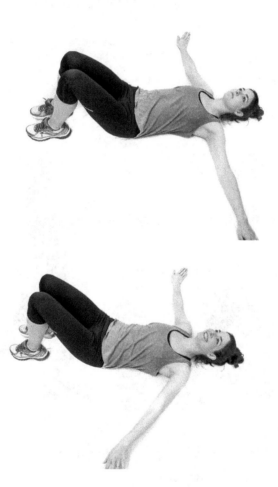

1. Lie on your back with your legs together, knees bent, and feet flat on the floor. Try to keep both arms and shoulders flat on the floor throughout the stretch.

2. Keeping your knees bent and together, slowly lower both legs to one side as far as you comfortably can.

3. Hold position for ten to thirty seconds.

4. Bring your legs back up slowly and repeat toward the other side.

5. Continue alternating sides for at least three to five times on each side.

CALF STRETCH

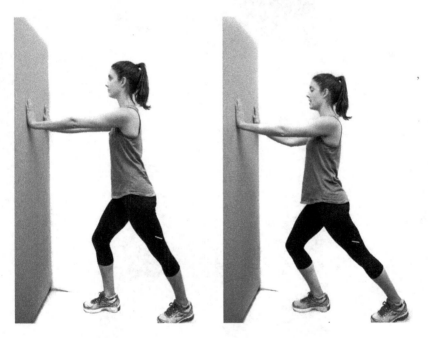

1. Stand facing a wall slightly farther than arm's length away, feet shoulder width apart.

2. Put your palms flat against the wall at shoulder height and shoulder width apart.

3. Step forward with your right leg and bend your right knee. Keeping both feet flat on the floor, bend your left knee slightly until you feel a stretch in your left calf muscle. It shouldn't feel uncomfortable. If you don't feel a stretch, bend your right knee until you do.

4. Hold position for ten to thirty seconds and then return to the starting position.

5. Repeat with your left leg.

6. Continue alternating legs for at least three to five times each leg.

Strength-Training Exercises

Strength training builds muscle. When you begin your strength training, choose weights or a resistance level that will allow you to do two sets of ten repetitions. When that becomes too easy, increase the weight or resistance. With respect to weight-bearing exercises (push-ups, planks, squats, etc.), start with two sets of one or two repetitions and work your way up to two sets of ten.

Try to do strength-training exercises for all of your major muscle groups on two or more days per week for thirty minutes at a time, but don't exercise the same muscle group on any two days in a row.

The six strength-training exercises shown below target the upper and lower body.

UPPER BODY EXERCISES

1. Arm curls

2. Side arm raises

3. Chair dips

LOWER BODY EXERCISES

1. Back leg raises

2. Leg straightening exercises

3. Toe stands

ARM CURLS

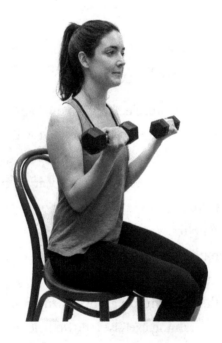

1. Stand or sit with your feet shoulder width apart.

2. Hold the weights straight down at your sides, palms facing forward. Breathe in slowly.

3. Breathe out as you slowly bend your elbows and lift the weights toward your chest. Keep your elbows at your sides.

4. Hold the position for one second.

5. Breathe in as you slowly lower your arms.

6. Repeat ten to fifteen times.

7. Rest, then repeat ten to fifteen more times.

SIDE ARM RAISES

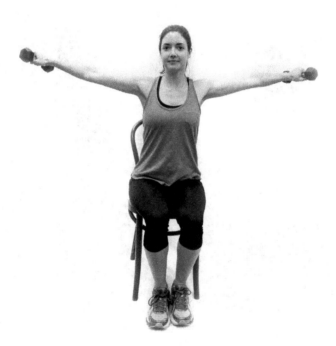

1. Stand or sit in a sturdy, armless chair.

2. Keep your feet flat on the floor, shoulder width apart.

3. Hold hand weights straight down at your sides with your palms facing inward.

4. Slowly breathe out as you raise both arms up to the side, shoulder height.

5. Hold the position for one second.

6. Breathe in as you slowly lower your arms to your sides.

7. Repeat ten to fifteen times.

8. Rest, then repeat ten to fifteen more times.

CHAIR DIPS

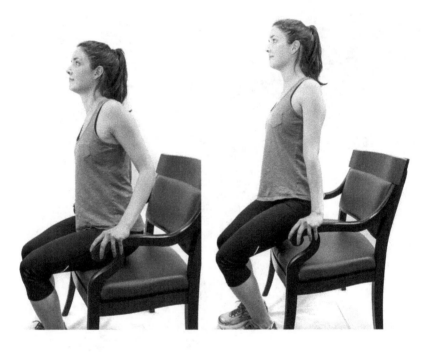

1. Sit in a sturdy chair with armrests with your feet flat on the floor, shoulder width apart.

2. Lean slightly forward; keep your back and shoulders straight.

3. Grasp the arms of the chair with your hands next to you. Breathe in slowly.

4. Breathe out and use your arms to push your body slowly off the chair.

5. Hold position for one second.

6. Breathe in as you slowly lower yourself back down.

7. Repeat ten to fifteen times.

8. Rest, then repeat ten to fifteen more times.

BACK LEG RAISES

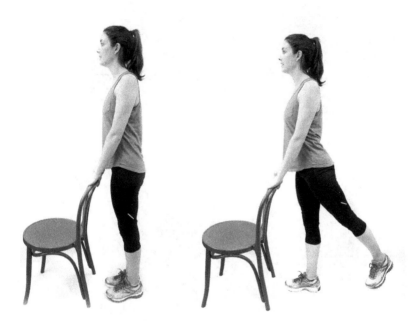

1. Hold on to the back of a sturdy chair or counter for balance. Breathe in slowly.

2. Breathe out and slowly lift one leg straight back without bending your knee or pointing your toes. Try not to lean forward. The leg you are standing on should be slightly bent.

3. Hold position for one second.

4. Breathe in as you slowly lower your leg.

5. Repeat ten to fifteen times.

6. Repeat ten to fifteen times with other leg.

7. Repeat ten to fifteen more times with each leg.

LEG STRENGTHENING EXERCISES

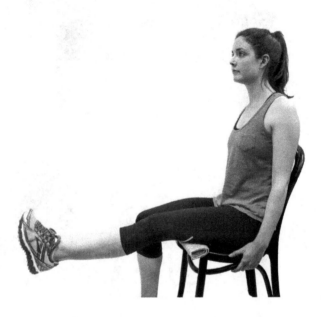

1. Sit in a sturdy chair with your back supported by the chair. Only the balls of your feet and your toes should rest on the floor.

2. Put a rolled bath towel at the edge of the chair under thighs for support.

3. Breathe in slowly.

4. Breathe out and slowly extend one leg in front of you as straight as possible, but don't lock your knee.

5. Flex foot to point toes toward the ceiling. Hold position for one second.

6. Breathe in as you slowly lower leg back down.

7. Repeat ten to fifteen times.

8. Repeat ten to fifteen times with other leg.

9. Repeat ten to fifteen more times with each leg.

TOE STANDS

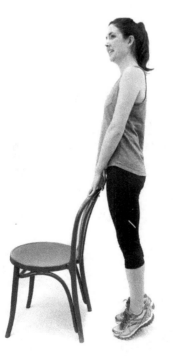

1. Stand behind a sturdy chair, feet shoulder width apart, holding on for balance. Breathe in slowly.

2. Breathe out and slowly stand on tiptoes, as high as possible.

3. Hold position for one second.

4. Breathe in as you slowly lower heels to the floor.

5. Repeat ten to fifteen times.

6. Rest, then repeat ten to fifteen more times.

As noted earlier, these exercises are provided as a general guide to get you started on an exercise routine. Depending on your level of fitness, you may want to engage in a more challenging set of exercises. The American Heart Association's website (heart.org) is a great resource with helpful information about fitness and tips on how to stay active.

Recover

RX FOR HEART ATTACK SURVIVORS

If you have survived a heart attack, you have a lot to be thankful for! Over the past two decades, significant advances have been made in diagnosing and treating women with heart disease. The combination of awareness and treatment is estimated to save the lives of more than three hundred women who suffer from all forms of heart disease *every day*. We call this secondary prevention.

If you have survived a heart attack, you may still be scared, confused, or worried about making certain lifestyle changes and perhaps adding new medications to your daily routine. If you don't make changes in your life and address what put you at risk of heart attack in the first place, you are in danger of having another

> OVER THE PAST TWO DECADES, SIGNIFICANT ADVANCES HAVE BEEN MADE IN DIAGNOSING AND TREATING WOMEN WITH HEART DISEASE.

one. Now is the time to start over and follow the advice we have given you to stay on the road to good health.

This chapter provides information relevant to women who have already had a heart attack. Even if you haven't suffered one yourself, you may wish to continue reading to help or support a friend or loved one who has. After a heart attack, you may worry about resuming regular daily activities or adhering to the rules of healthy living. But there is nothing to worry about. You can do this if you focus on making small but consistent changes to the way you live.

Healing after Open-Heart Surgery

If your surgery left you with an incision on your chest along the breastbone (sternum), wait for the bone and skin to heal before you resume normal activities. This takes anywhere from six to ten weeks. You will likely be seeing your heart surgeon for regular follow-ups in the first two to three months after your operation, and the surgeon will inform you when your sternum has healed.

Even after the skin is healed and the breastbone has knitted completely, this area can remain sensitive for a while, so you may need to be creative in terms of your clothing, undergarments, sleeping position, and routine activities of living, including sexual activity and positions (see "Yes, Sex!" below). This is temporary! Once the breastbone is totally healed, these issues should not be of further concern.

If you have any reservations, talk to your doctor.

The Importance of Cardiac Rehabilitation

Whether you had a heart attack, underwent a stent placement, had open heart surgery, or discovered that your shortness of breath was related to heart failure, your doctor will likely recommend you enroll in a cardiac rehabilitation program. Cardiac rehab is designed specifically to help you recover after a heart procedure, heart attack, or hospitalization or even stop the progression of the disease after a new diagnosis of certain heart conditions. Cardiac rehab has been shown to decrease mortality rates, reduce symptoms of heart disease, and decrease hospital readmissions.

Cardiac rehabilitation and other secondary prevention programs have been developed to protect against the recurrence of heart attacks through graduated physical activity and muscle training. This physical training along with education and counseling will provide you with a better understanding of your condition along with practical ways to eat healthier and manage stress, anger, and depression—all common factors in heart disease. Cardiac rehab programs are especially valuable—and underused by women! A coordinated team of doctors, nurses, and physical therapists runs these programs, many of which also offer the services of dieticians and behavioral health professionals, as well as access to integrative health modalities like yoga and tai chi.

GETTING INTO A CARDIAC REHAB PROGRAM

Referral to cardiac rehab should be discussed with your doctor at the time of your heart event. You may need to wait for several weeks to months before it is safe to begin, and you will likely require a stress test to assess your ideal exercise prescription. Rehab sessions are usually two to three times each week for a minimum of twelve weeks. The program will be customized for you and take into account your physical activity prior to your heart event, your degree of physical stamina, and medical facts about your heart, along with the findings from your stress test. Physical activity will be monitored initially to check your EKG, heart rate, and blood pressure, along with any symptoms you may feel (such as chest pain, breathlessness, or leg fatigue). Your program will gradually increase in intensity and duration of exercise while you are being monitored. This approach allows you to safely learn the ideal way for you to stay physically active in the future. The careful monitoring, too, has been shown to be an effective way to help women increase their confidence and minimize their fears about being active. You'll take away from this rehab experience the knowledge to help you understand the importance of staying active and the wherewithal to do it on your own after the program is finished.

MORE THAN JUST EXERCISE

Cardiac rehab programs also include nutritional education and access to behavioral health professionals and other programs to optimize recovery. For example, there may be group sessions for stress management or a one-on-one evaluation with a psychologist or psychiatrist, because new research has confirmed what we have suspected: that stress, depression, and feelings of anger can increase the risk of heart disease recurrence.

Cardiac rehab programs also include help for stopping smoking, referrals to sleep programs for those with sleep disorders, and social support from other women.

Yes, Sex!

Sex is a subject on the mind of every heart patient. Whether you have had open-heart surgery or a heart attack, we're sure you are wondering when you can resume sexual activity—or even *if* you can. The good news is that sex, like any other physical activity, will again be part of your life. Unless your doctor tells you otherwise, you can resume sexual activity when you feel comfortable doing it. Start slowly, and if anything bothers you or you feel physically uncomfortable, stop—just as you would when doing any exercise or even when climbing stairs! And just as with starting any new exercise, report any new or unusual symptoms, such as chest pain, palpitations, or breathlessness, to your doctor.

After open-heart surgery, be the less active partner and avoid placing any pressure on your chest or breastbone. Remember, this is temporary. You will know when you are ready to resume your normal sexual positions.

Communication with your partner is crucial! Discuss your feelings and fears before resuming your sex life. Your partner probably has the same concerns. Talk them out, work around them, and do not let them evolve into a stressful situation. Sex should be fun and should relieve stress—not cause it.

The Link between Depression, Anxiety, and Heart Disease

Behavioral cardiology is a relatively new area of research focusing on better understanding the link between our hearts and behavioral health. But one thing is for sure—if you are feeling sad, angry, or anxious after your heart event, you are not alone. Studies now prove a strong link between depression, anxiety, and heart disease in women. Not only are women who are depressed twice as likely to have heart problems (even if they don't have any other risk factors), but women with coronary heart disease who are depressed are twice as likely to suffer a fatal heart attack. It's also true that depression makes it more difficult to control blood pressure, which is crucial to preventing a heart attack.

More than 50 percent of women say they suffer from depression, anxiety, or both as a result of their heart disease, which helps explain why so few women actually make lifestyle changes after experiencing a heart event. If you are depressed or anxious, you are unlikely to have the incentive or energy to make the changes necessary to prevent another event, and this can also lead to nonadherence to prescribed medications or follow-up doctor appointments.

If you find yourself feeling this way, do not suffer in silence. Call your doctor as soon as possible. When you are recuperating from a heart attack, your emotional health is as important as your physical health. So ask for help.

Depression and anxiety are medical conditions that are absolutely treatable and respond to a combination of medication and counseling. Do not try to fight them alone! Speak with your doctor about your symptoms, which may include anger, sadness, anxiety, lack of interest in pleasurable activities, or significant changes in sleeping or eating patterns. This will be the first step toward getting your life back on track.

Even if you don't feel up to it, try to reach out to your friends and family. Stay in touch with a phone call or a note and maintain your social contacts. Having a strong support system improves survival in depressed women with heart disease. Your well-being and optimal recuperation depend on it. Help is available—but you need to ask for it!

WHERE TO GET HELP

Talk to your friends and family about heart disease. Explain to them what it is and talk about what you are going through. Some of the lifestyle changes you will be making will be easier if you have others understanding and participating with you. Collect brochures at the doctor's office, or request information from the American Heart Association (www.heart.org).

Get professional help. Reach out to your doctor or other clinicians for a referral or recommendation that is right for you.

Check out support groups. Sometimes it helps to talk to others who are experiencing the same thing you are, and support groups can help you connect with other women who suffer from heart disease. Your doctor will be able to suggest those in your area. You may also want to get connected with WomenHeart (www.womenheart.org), a national patient-centered organization dedicated to serving women with heart disease.

Take medication as prescribed. If your doctor has prescribed antidepressants, always take them as prescribed. Remember that, in general, these medications do not work immediately but may take several weeks for optimal effect. For the majority of women, it is the combination of counseling and medication that is most effective in fighting depression.

Exercise

Maintaining an exercise program is important in warding off heart disease, and it's equally important in preventing a second heart attack. Reread Week 2 of the Six S.T.E.P.S. in Six Weeks Program and get moving every day. If you have concerns because of your heart attack or recovery from surgery and you aren't sure about how much to exercise or what types of exercise you should be doing, talk to your doctor about cardiac rehab. Your insurance may even cover it. With rehab, you will gain the confidence you need to get more physically active and have the added benefit of meeting others who are fighting the same medical issues. Statistics show that women not only benefit greatly from cardiac rehabilitation but also go on to have a better quality of life than before their heart attack.

It's worth repeating that it's never too late to start being more physically active. If you don't know where to start, refer back to Week 2 of the program for some guidelines. You don't need to join a gym, but at the very least, take a short daily walk and then walk longer and longer distances or perhaps go a bit faster as you get stronger. Walking is great exercise because it's aerobic and increases your heart rate, which has been shown to decrease the incidence of heart disease and stroke. Brisk walking has further been shown to decrease incidence of a heart attack and death from heart disease in women. You can try one of the strength and flexibility exercises in the previous chapter. If you prefer other types of aerobic exercise, like swimming, jogging, running, or bicycling, great. Just check with your doctor before you start.

The bottom line is that physical activity keeps your heart and your bones healthy and strong, so *get moving*!

Take Your Medications

Be sure you are clear about *all* of the medications you are taking. This means knowing the name of every one, the dosage, the possible side effects, and the proper time of day to take them. Properly taking the medications prescribed by your doctor can make a huge difference in your overall health and your ability to recuperate and prevent a second attack. If you have concerns about any of your prescriptions, talk to your doctor or pharmacist, and never stop taking any of them on your own without consulting your doctor. It can actually be dangerous to stop some medications abruptly. If you think you are having side effects from one or more of your meds, be sure to report these concerns to your doctor immediately. If the cost of your medications is an issue, mention this as well; there are often less expensive alternatives that your doctor can prescribe.

ASPIRIN

Studies show that for women who have had a heart attack, low-dose aspirin (81 mg) taken daily helps to lower the risk of having another one, with the added benefit of preventing stroke. Aspirin also helps keep the arteries open in women who have had heart bypass or other procedures, such as coronary angioplasty. Taking aspirin regularly is particularly important if you had a stent placed after a heart attack; you should never stop taking it unless you are told to do so by your cardiologist. For some people, taking aspirin can have risks, especially if you have had serious bleeding in the past, so be sure to tell your doctor if this pertains to you.

Recent studies have shown there is no benefit for daily aspirin in most women without known heart disease. This is something of a change from prior recommendations, so please be sure to check with your doctor before starting or stopping daily aspirin use.

Be careful not to confuse aspirin with other common over-the-counter pain-relieving products, such as acetaminophen (Tylenol), ibuprofen (Advil, Motrin), or naproxen sodium (Aleve). These products are all effective for treating pain and fever, but only aspirin has been demonstrated to be beneficial in preventing stroke or recurrent heart attack. If you are taking aspirin, do not take any of the above medications unless your doctor approves. Always remember to tell your doctor about all medications you take, even those that are over the counter.

HORMONE REPLACEMENT THERAPY
AND ORAL CONTRACEPTION

The American Heart Association does *not* recommend that hormone replacement therapy (HRT) be given to prevent heart disease; it *does* recommend that *any* woman who smokes, has heart disease or high blood pressure, or has suffered a stroke should *not take hormones.*

If you were taking HRT by mouth at the time of your heart event, talk with your doctor about how to safely discontinue use. Do not stop on your own or all at once. Topical estrogens, on the other hand, can be used even by many women with heart disease to decrease symptoms of vaginal dryness, but their use should be discussed with your doctor.

For some women who suffer symptoms (significant mood swings, sleep issues, hot flashes) in the perimenopause and menopause period, consideration for short-term HRT use, ideally started soon after your periods stop, may be an option. Be sure to discuss these issues and concerns with your doctor. Women who take oral contraceptives should review any potential health issues with their doctors on a regular basis.

See the Dentist Regularly

Gum disease (gingivitis and periodontal disease) can make you almost twice as likely to suffer from coronary artery disease. This may be because there is increased inflammation from even mild periodontal disease or because bacteria in the mouth enter the bloodstream and worsen the plaque growing on the artery walls.

What's more, active gum disease can worsen an existing heart condition by causing infective endocarditis. If your dentist and cardiologist determine your heart problem puts you at risk, then one of them will prescribe antibiotics for you to take before all dental procedures. Be sure to take these antibiotics as prescribed before every visit to a dentist, even for simple teeth cleanings!

Protect your heart by practicing good oral hygiene. Brush twice a day and floss every night before bed. Also make sure to have your teeth cleaned regularly, one to four times a year, as prescribed by your dentist.

Choose to Be Happy

When we feel good, we are happy and optimistic about the future. If you don't feel this way most days or if you often wake up stressed out or worried, your health can be affected. Although some of us are naturally more happy or optimistic, we can all choose to be happier. The science of happiness has received a great deal of attention over the past decade, and we know that there are skills we can practice to lead toward living a happier and more optimistic life.

Of course, we all have our off days, weeks, and even months, but if you feel stressed, sad, or pessimistic about the future, then you need to do something. Start with reaching out to friends, family, and perhaps your doctor.

Don't assume the worst. You may just need a little emotional or psychological tune-up. Maybe it's time to resume a hobby that once gave you joy. Get out of the house and enjoy a movie, go to dinner, or listen to some music. See some friends. Do anything you can to bring joy into your life. Perhaps what you need to do is knock a few things off your to-do list and have more time for yourself. Even having an extra ten minutes a day to do absolutely nothing can be a help. It is just as important to make time for doing the activities that bring you joy as it is to identify, minimize, or remove the stressors that make you unhappy.

Remember, as with all other lifestyle changes, it is not an all-or-nothing proposition. Some things that are stressful simply cannot be avoided, just as most of us are not able to enjoy endless leisure activities. But the important thing is to give yourself the choice to be happier by changing what you can.

There are many excellent resources that will guide you as you begin to practice healthy habits to help manage stress and experience more joy in your daily life. Check out the Mayo Clinic's website (mayoclinic.org) or that of the Harvard Medical School (health. harvard.edu) for additional strategies and techniques you can use to enhance your health and well-being.

Trust Your Intuition

We have heard many women say that they had a sense that something just wasn't right before they suffered a heart attack. There is something to that. If you suspect something isn't as it should be, trust your gut instinct—your woman's intuition. We have been around a long time, have seen enough patients, and have heard enough stories to know that acting on a strong hunch can be a lifesaver. Also, don't be afraid to get a second or even a third opinion if you feel any doctor is not taking your complaint seriously or minimizing your symptoms. If you continue to feel something's not right, find a doctor who will listen and will be responsive to your concerns.

Heal

COMMON HEART MEDICATIONS, TREATMENTS, AND TESTS

Once heart disease has developed, or if you are making an effort to reduce your risk of developing heart disease when risk factors are present, there are several treatment options, beginning with various types of medications. Some medicines decrease the workload on the heart, while others reduce the chance of having a heart attack or dying suddenly. Still others prevent or delay the need for a special procedure, such as angioplasty or bypass surgery. Several types of medicine are commonly used.

Medications

ACEIs (angiotensin-converting enzyme inhibitors) help to lower blood pressure and reduce strain on your heart. They may also reduce the risk of a future heart attack and heart failure. Commonly used ACE inhibitors include benazepril (Lotensin), captopril (Capoten), enalapril (Vasotec), lisinopril (Prinivil, Zestril), and ramipril (Altace).

ARBs (angiotensin-receptor blocking agents) are similar to ACEIs in their indications for use and protective effects for those with hypertension, heart failure, or even kidney disease. ARBs are less likely to result in the side effect of a cough, which can be seen with ACEIs. Commonly used ARBs include losartan (Cozaar), valsartan (Diovan), candesartan (Atacand), and telmisartan (Micardis).

Anticoagulants help to prevent clots from forming in your arteries and blocking blood flow. In certain abnormal heart rhythms, they may be prescribed to decrease the risk of stroke. A commonly used anticoagulant is warfarin (Coumadin).

Novel oral anticoagulants (NOACs), also known as direct oral anticoagulants (DOACs), are newer agents that are used for similar indications as traditional anticoagulants but do not require regular blood tests to monitor dosing. These include dabigatran (Pradaxa), apixaban (Eliquis), and rivaroxaban (Xarelto).

Aspirin and other antiplatelet agents help prevent clots from forming in your arteries and blocking blood flow. Aspirin may not be appropriate for some people, because it increases the risk of bleeding. Other antiplatelet agents that may be combined with aspirin include ticagrelor (Brilinta), prasugrel (Effient), and clopidogrel (Plavix).

Beta-blockers slow your heart rate and lower your blood pressure to decrease the workload on your heart. They are used to relieve angina and may also reduce the risk of a future heart attack. They have also been found effective in treating heart failure. Commonly used beta-blockers are atenolol (Tenormin), metoprolol (Lopressor), propranolol (Inderal), and carvedilol (Coreg).

Calcium channel blockers relax blood vessels and lower blood pressure, ease the heart's workload, help widen coronary arteries, and relieve and control angina. They may also treat common causes of palpitations. Commonly used medications are amlodipine (Norvasc), verapamil (Calan), diltiazem (Cardizem), and nifedipine (Procardia).

Cholesterol-lowering medicines help to reduce your cholesterol to a doctor-recommended level. Commonly used cholesterol-lowering medications are the statins: simvastatin (Zocor), atorvastatin (Lipitor), rosuvastatin (Crestor), and pravastatin (Pravachol). Ezetimibe (Zetia) may be added to a statin for increased lipid lowering. Elevated triglycerides can be treated with gemfibrozil (Lopid) or fenofibrate (Tricor).

Newer lipid-lowering agents, called PCSK9 inhibitors, were developed for those who cannot tolerate statin drugs or for whom statins do not sufficiently lower the cholesterol levels: evolocumab (Repatha) and alirocumab (Praluent). These medications are given by self-injection every two to four weeks.

Long-acting nitrates are similar to nitroglycerin but are longer acting and can limit the occurrence of chest pain when used regularly over a long period. Commonly used nitrates are isosorbide dinitrate (Isordil) and isosorbide mononitrate (Imdur). One agent for those who continue to have chest pain despite the use of several medications is ranolazine (Ranexa).

A recent clinical research study showed that Black patients with heart failure who take a fixed-dose combination of the medications isosorbide dinitrate and hydralazine (BiDil) had significantly decreased deaths from heart failure.

Nitroglycerin widens the coronary arteries, increasing blood flow to the heart muscle and relieving chest pain. Nitroglycerin sublingual (NTG-SL) tablets are small tablets that are placed under the tongue in the setting of acute chest pain.

Diuretics are used to lower blood pressure and can be helpful for patients with heart failure. They include furosemide (Lasix), chlorthalidone (Hygroton), and hydrochlorothiazide (HCTZ).

NEWER HEART MEDICATIONS

New classes of drugs that treat type 2 diabetes have been shown to be helpful to prevent heart attack and improve heart failure. These are known as SGLT-2 inhibitors. They include dapagliflozin (Farxiga), empagliflozin (Jardiance), and canagliflozin (Invokana). Another class of newer drugs called GLP-1 receptor agonists include liraglutide (Victoza), semaglutide (Ozempic), and dulaglutide (Trulicity).

Newer classes of heart failure drugs that prevent hospitalization have recently been approved. These include sacubitril/valsartan (Entresto).

> NEW CLASSES OF DRUGS THAT TREAT TYPE 2 DIABETES HAVE BEEN SHOWN TO BE HELPFUL TO PREVENT HEART ATTACK AND IMPROVE HEART FAILURE.

Invasive or Surgical Treatments

Surgery or a cardiac intervention, along with optimal medication use, may be indicated in certain clinical situations and may be more effective in managing symptoms and even in prolonging life. These treatments (angioplasty, stenting, and bypass surgery) may be used to treat coronary artery disease if medications and lifestyle changes haven't improved symptoms or if blockages are numerous and very severe.

Angioplasty opens blocked or narrowed coronary arteries, improving blood flow to the heart, relieving chest pain, and possibly preventing a heart attack. Sometimes a device called a stent is placed in the artery to keep the artery open after the procedure.

During **coronary artery bypass surgery**, arteries or veins are taken from other places in your body to bypass narrowed coronary arteries. Bypass surgery can improve blood flow to the heart, relieve chest pain, and prevent a heart attack.

Your doctor may prescribe **cardiac rehabilitation** for angina or after bypass surgery, angioplasty, a heart attack, or worsening symptoms of heart failure. Cardiac rehab can help you recover faster, feel better, and develop a healthier lifestyle. Almost everyone with coronary artery disease can benefit from cardiac rehab. Rehab usually includes exercise training, education about nutrition, stress management, and other ways to live a healthier life.

Tests

Although we presented a heart disease "risk assessment" at the beginning of this book, there really isn't a standard heart disease test. If your doctor suspects heart disease, you will be asked about your medical history and your family's health. Next, the doctor will check to see if you have any risk factors and perform a physical exam. Based on the results of these preliminary procedures, your doctor may order an electrocardiogram (EKG), an echocardiogram, a stress test, or other diagnostic tests. These tests fall into two categories: noninvasive and invasive.

NONINVASIVE TESTS

Blood tests may be ordered by your doctor, including a fasting glucose test or a test called hemoglobin A1c (Hgb A1c) to check your blood sugar level and a fasting lipoprotein profile to check your cholesterol levels. These tests can identify modifiable risk factors for cardiovascular disease.

A **chest X-ray** takes a picture of the organs and structures inside the chest, including the heart, lungs, and blood vessels.

An **EKG** (electrocardiogram) measures the rate and regularity of your heartbeat, identifies prior heart attacks, and checks for heart muscle thickening related to long-standing hypertension.

Stress tests are often used to diagnose when your heart is working harder and beating faster than when it is at rest. During exercise stress testing, your blood pressure and EKG readings are monitored while you walk or run on a treadmill or pedal a bicycle. For certain people, stress testing is combined with heart imaging.

Heart-imaging tests can be performed at rest to evaluate the structure of the heart, or they can be combined with exercise or medications that cause the heart to be "stressed" to answer questions about the presence of artery blockages or risk of heart attack.

Echocardiography uses sound waves to show the heart's structure, blood flow through the chambers, and the strength of the heart muscle.

A **nuclear heart scan** uses a radioactive tracer and a special camera to evaluate the blood flow to the heart during exercise and at rest. A nuclear scan can find scar tissue indicating that a heart attack occurred.

A **CT scan of the heart** is a newer heart-imaging test that can be combined with a calcium artery score to provide noninvasive images of the coronary arteries and also to provide information about the beginnings of plaque formation in the arteries.

An **MRI of the heart** is also a newer heart-imaging test; it provides additional information about the heart's structure and function.

INVASIVE TESTS

Cardiac catheterization (coronary angiography) can identify problems with the arteries of the heart. A thin plastic tube is passed through an artery in the groin or arm to reach the coronary arteries. A special dye is injected into the tube so X-rays can show whether there is any artery blockage or other heart problems.

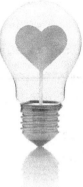

Q&A about Heart Disease

As you build your heart knowledge, you will undoubtedly have questions—questions about your risk factors, questions about the safety of certain medications or activities. On the pages that follow, we share some of the questions we're asked most often by women. But these are only a first step; we encourage you to write down your questions and share them with your healthcare provider, who can provide answers and recommendations specific to you.

Q. I was diagnosed with gestational diabetes during my second and third pregnancy, but this resolved after each delivery. Am I at risk for diabetes in the future? At risk for heart disease?

A. Recent research has shown that issues during pregnancy, including high blood pressure, gestational diabetes, preeclampsia, eclampsia, and babies born very small or very large, are considered to be risk factors for future heart disease. Some have called these clinical conditions "failed stress tests" of pregnancy. They were included in the most recent guidelines on risk factors for heart disease in women. You should speak with your primary care doctor to see how to assess all your risks for heart disease and start early to minimize them. Women who have been diagnosed with gestational diabetes are also at significantly greater risk for developing type 2 diabetes within five to ten years after delivery.

Q. I recently had a heart attack, and I want to know when it is safe to return to sexual activity with my partner. Are there limitations?

A. Adjusting to life after a heart attack can be challenging, but we know that intimacy is an extremely important part of healing and living, so you should look at it as another physical activity you'll be resuming. The American Heart Association has released recommendations about sex and heart disease. Unless your doctor tells you otherwise, you may resume sexual activity as soon as you feel comfortable. Always start slowly, and if you become uncomfortable, stop—just as you would when climbing stairs! If you are postmenopausal and suffer from vaginal dryness leading to painful intercourse, it is probably safe to use topical estrogen cream, but check with your doctor.

If you have had heart surgery and have an incision on your chest along the breastbone, you need to allow the bone and skin incision to heal. Sexual activity can be resumed slowly; you just need to be a bit more creative in terms of activities and positions, so take it easy. It's also best to be the less active partner during sex and try to avoid placing pressure on your chest or breastbone.

Communication with your partner is crucial! Before resuming sexual activity, talk about your feelings and fears. Your partner most likely has the same fears and concerns that you do.

Q. I was diagnosed with lupus as a young adult. I have read about the link between inflammation and heart disease. Am I at higher risk because of my long-standing lupus?

A. Along with pregnancy-related conditions, rheumatologic diseases like lupus, rheumatoid arthritis, and scleroderma are also risk factors for heart disease. These conditions are much more common in women than in men and have been shown to increase the risk of heart disease and stroke.

It is likely that the inflammatory abnormalities seen in these diseases cause inflammatory changes in blood vessels that lead to a higher risk of disease. Also, some of the medications used to treat these conditions, like steroids or prednisone, may increase the risk.

Q. Is it safe to take an aspirin a day to prevent heart disease?

A. If you've already had a heart attack, low-dose aspirin (81 mg daily) helps to lower the risk of having another one, and recent studies also have shown that low-dose aspirin prevents stroke in women. Aspirin also helps to keep arteries open if you have had a heart bypass or other artery-opening procedure, such as coronary angioplasty. However, aspirin may be harmful for some people, especially those with gastrointestinal conditions like ulcer disease. Talk to your doctor about whether taking aspirin is right for you. Be sure not to confuse aspirin with other common pain-relieving products such as acetaminophen (Tylenol), ibuprofen (Advil, Motrin), and naproxen sodium (Aleve). For some women with known heart disease, nonsteroidal anti-inflammatory drugs like ibuprofen may in fact be harmful. Be sure to tell your doctor about all your medications, including vitamins and other over-the-counter agents.

Q. I know that stress isn't good for you, but are behavioral issues really related to heart disease?

A. We have long known that stress can be harmful, but there is more and more data that shows the harmful effects of stress, depression, and even insufficient sleep in relation to heart disease. We also know that stress-reducing activities—yoga, mindfulness, cognitive behavior therapy—have a positive effect on heart health. And the importance of six to eight hours of sleep each night is clearly related to improved health.

Q. I heard that people with gum disease are at risk for heart disease. Is that true?

A. It's true. Researchers have found that people with gum disease are almost twice as likely to suffer from coronary artery disease as those without periodontal disease. There are several theories. First, many scientists believe that bacteria in the mouth can affect the heart by entering the bloodstream, attaching to fatty plaque in the heart blood vessels and contributing to clot formation. Coronary artery disease is characterized by a thickening of the walls of the coronary arteries due to the buildup of cholesterol and other fatty compounds, calcium, and additional inflammatory substances. Blood clots can obstruct normal blood flow, restricting the amount of nutrients and oxygen required for the heart to function properly. This may lead to heart attacks. Another possibility is that the inflammation caused by periodontal disease increases plaque buildup, which may contribute to swelling of the arteries.

Periodontal disease also can worsen existing heart conditions. For example, patients at risk for infective endocarditis may require antibiotics before having any dental procedures. Your dentist and cardiologist will be able to determine whether your heart condition requires use of antibiotics prior to dental procedures. So practice good oral housekeeping: brush twice a day and floss once every day. Have your teeth cleaned at least once a year (every six months is better).

Q. Do birth control pills or hormone replacement therapy (HRT) increase a woman's risk for heart disease?

A. For the vast majority of women, the use of birth control pills is safe. But women over the age of thirty-five or those with other cardiovascular risk factors—in particular, smoking—should speak with their physicians to weigh the risks and benefits of taking birth control pills.

Recent studies have shown that women who have gone through menopause and who have heart disease may have a higher risk of another cardiac problem—such as a heart attack—after starting HRT, at least in the short term. Women who have had a stroke have a higher risk of another stroke if they start HRT.

However, new studies show that many women may be able to use HRT beginning at menopause for a short period of time to minimize the vasomotor effects of no longer getting their periods. Also, topical estrogen or vaginal estrogen can help with vaginal dryness.

Women should speak with their physicians to assess the risks versus benefits of HRT or other forms of estrogen replacement.

Q. Is it OK to take vitamins and herbs for heart problems?

A. When it comes to vitamins and herbs, it's always best to check with both your pharmacist and your doctor before adding them to your daily regimen. There is a common misconception that because a prescription isn't needed for vitamins and herbs, they're always safe to take. That is certainly not the case! All drugs, whether over the counter or prescription, can interact with each other—some in harmful ways. This is why communication with your doctor and pharmacist is crucial. It is important to bring along a written list of every drug, herb, supplement, and vitamin you are taking. Drug interactions may not show up on the pharmacy computer if the list of what you are taking is incomplete.

But yes, you can take vitamins and herbal remedies, if your doctor and pharmacist know about them to ensure that there are not any side effects. Be sure to take your prescription and nonprescription medications list along whenever you go to a doctor, dentist, surgeon, nurse practitioner, nutritionist, or hospital. Tell all of your providers what you are taking. It is your responsibility to do so. Only then can they provide the proper recommendations.

Q. I had open-heart surgery a few weeks ago. Why am I still so sad and tired?

A. Recent scientific studies have shown a strong link between depression and heart disease in women. Women who are depressed are twice as likely to suffer heart problems, even in the absence of other risk factors. Also, women with coronary heart disease are twice as likely to die if they show symptoms of depression. Depression also makes it harder to control blood pressure.

A very high percentage of women (more than half) say they suffer depression, anxiety, or both as a result of heart disease.

But depression is absolutely treatable and responds to a combination of medication and counseling more than 90 percent of the time. In addition, strong social support improves survival in depressed women with heart disease.

An important component of cardiac rehab and secondary prevention programs is a focus on minimizing depression and anxiety after a heart event. Women are less likely to attend cardiac rehab programs and are more likely to benefit from them! Ask your doctor how to find a cardiac rehab program in your area.

Depression can be conquered with a combination of social support, antidepressants, and therapy. Collect brochures from your doctor's office and get information from the American Heart Association or WomenHeart about living and coping with heart disease. Share this information with your family and friends so they know what to expect and how they can help in your recovery from a heart attack or surgery.

Support groups are key. If you've done all that you feel you're capable of and you're still feeling depressed, seek out professional help. Don't hesitate to ask your doctor for a recommendation. Check the WomenHeart website, www.womenheart.org, for a group in your neighborhood.

Q. What about going to rehab or a gym after a heart attack? My doctor never mentioned it. Is it too late now?

A. It is never too late to start exercise, and you don't need to join a gym to get the benefits of exercise on the heart. If you've had a heart attack or coronary heart surgery, cardiac rehabilitation is of great benefit and is usually covered by insurance. So ask your doctor and sign up! Studies have shown that after heart attacks and coronary heart surgery, women benefit from cardiac rehabilitation and have a better quality of life. Cardiac rehab programs also include important programs on nutrition, stress management, and other ways to lead a heart-healthy life after a cardiac event. These programs have been shown to decrease the risk of a second heart event.

Aerobic exercise—that is, exercise that increases your heart rate—such as walking, swimming, jogging, and running, has been shown to decrease the incidence of heart disease and stroke. Brisk walking has been shown to decrease the incidence of heart attacks and death from heart disease in women. Therefore, a simple goal of incorporating walking into your daily life could help to prevent a heart attack.

Recent guidelines suggest 150 minutes of moderate-intensity activity each week or 75 minutes of high-intensity activity. Also, remember to do resistance training (light weights) and stretching regularly.

Q. I had breast cancer ten years ago and was treated with a combination of chemotherapy and radiation therapy. I have been cancer-free ever since but am wondering if this prior treatment has put my heart at risk.

A. Radiation therapy, as well as other types of cancer treatment, can present an increased risk of heart disease. If you are a cancer survivor who has had chemotherapy, radiation, or any combination thereof, it is of the utmost importance to maintain a healthy lifestyle by following our Six S.T.E.P.S. program. Exercise, maintaining a healthy weight, controlling blood pressure, and preventing diabetes all positively impact the body's ability to compensate for the bodily stress of chemotherapy and radiation. Based on your type of treatment, certain cardiac testing may be recommended.

If you are about to embark upon a cancer treatment protocol, partnering with your oncologist and your cardiologist is essential to ensure the optimal combination and dose of therapies to maximize effectiveness in treating the cancer while also minimizing your risks of developing heart disease.

Women with preexisting cardiac risk factors such as obesity, diabetes, high blood pressure, family history, etc. are at an even greater risk of developing heart disease after cancer treatment. For those women, adhering to a heart-healthy lifestyle is critical.

Q. I was recently diagnosed with lupus, an autoimmune disease. In assessing my risk factor profile, autoimmune diseases are included in the "modifiable" category. I don't understand this categorization, since this autoimmune disease will always be present and part of my overall health profile. Can you explain this?

A. As a general rule, risk factors that are considered "modifiable" are those that, once diagnosed (e.g., diabetes, autoimmune diseases, etc.), can have the inherent risk related to heart disease modified with appropriate treatment. Nonmodifiable risk factors such as family history or age cannot be "improved upon" in any way.

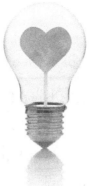

Glossary

Aerobic exercise. Sustained exercise such as jogging, cycling, or swimming that stimulates and strengthens the heart and lungs, thereby improving the body's utilization of oxygen.

Angina. Chest pain caused by a shortage of blood and oxygen to the heart.

Angioplasty. A procedure in which a device with a small balloon on the tip of a catheter is inserted into a blood vessel to open up a blocked area. Often angioplasty procedures include the placement of a stent and are referred to as "percutaneous cardiac interventions."

Anticoagulants. Drugs used to prevent the formation of blood clots.

Antigen. A substance recognized as foreign by the immune system.

Aorta. The body's main artery, bringing oxygenated blood from the left side of the heart to the body.

Arrhythmia. An abnormal heart rhythm.

Arteriogram. An X-ray of the arteries that uses a special dye that can detect blockage or narrowing of the vessels. Also called an angiogram.

Artery. Blood vessel that carries blood from the heart to other parts of the body.

Atherosclerosis. A condition in which the artery walls thicken and narrow due to the buildup of cholesterol, restricting blood flow and leading to a heart attack, stroke, or damage to other vital organs, such as kidneys. Also referred to as arteriosclerosis.

Atria. The heart's two upper chambers. The right atrium receives blood returning to the heart from the body. The left atrium receives oxygenated blood from the lungs.

Atrial fibrillation. Irregular beating of the left or right upper chamber of the heart when electrical signals are fired in a very fast and uncontrolled manner.

Atypical chest pain. A term that is no longer recommended to describe pain that is not likely to be due to heart disease. The recommended term is "noncardiac chest pain."

Autoimmune diseases. A varied group of illnesses that involve almost every human organ system, including the nervous, gastrointestinal, and endocrine systems, as well as skin and other connective tissues, eyes, blood, and blood vessels. The body's immune system becomes misdirected and attacks the very organs it was designed to protect. Autoimmune diseases include systemic lupus erythematosus, rheumatoid arthritis, and Sjögren's syndrome. These diseases affect women three times more than men and are linked to an increased risk for heart disease.

Body mass index (BMI). A measure of body fat based on height and weight that applies to adult men and women. BMI categories: underweight = <18.5; normal weight = 18.5–24.9; overweight = 25–29.9; obese = 30 or greater.

Capillary. Thin-walled tube that carries blood between arteries and veins.

Cardiac arrest. A condition in which the heart stops beating and, if not treated immediately, can result in death.

Cardiac catheterization. A procedure that examines the heart structure by passing a thin tube into the heart through a vein or artery to evaluate pressures and oxygen levels and to assess chamber function.

Cardiac perfusion imaging. A noninvasive diagnostic procedure in which a small dose of radioactive fluid is injected into the bloodstream and collects in the wall of the heart, used to assess the heart's blood flow or heart attack damage.

Cardiology. A branch of medicine dealing with the heart and circulatory system.

Cardiomyopathy. A disease of the heart muscle in which the heart loses its ability to pump blood appropriately.

Cardiopulmonary resuscitation (CPR). A technique used in an emergency when breathing has stopped or a heart has stopped beating.

Cardiovascular. Pertaining to the heart and blood vessels.

Cardiovascular disease (CVD). Any abnormal condition of the heart or blood vessels, including coronary heart disease, stroke, congestive heart failure, peripheral vascular disease, congenital heart disease, endocarditis, and many other conditions.

Cardiovascular system. The heart, blood vessels, and blood transported by the blood vessels.

Carotid arteries. The arteries located on either side of the neck that supply the brain with blood.

Carotid endarterectomy. Surgery used to remove plaque from the carotid arteries.

Cholesterol. A waxy substance produced naturally by the liver that circulates in the blood and helps maintain tissues and cell membranes. Cholesterol is found throughout the body, including the nervous system, muscles, skin, liver, intestines, and heart. Too much cholesterol can contribute to atherosclerosis and other forms of cardiovascular disease.

Computed tomography (CT or CAT scan). Detailed images of internal organs obtained by taking a series of X-ray images from different angles. Computer processing is used to create cross-sectional images or "slices" of the bones, blood vessels, and soft tissues inside the body.

Coronary arteries. Blood vessels that receive oxygenated blood from the aorta and branch off into a network of smaller arteries that feed blood directly to the heart muscle.

Coronary artery disease (CAD). A condition caused by narrowed coronary arteries (atherosclerosis) that decreases the supply of blood to the heart (myocardial ischemia). Also known as ischemic heart disease.

Diabetes (diabetes mellitus). A group of diseases that results in too much sugar in the blood.

Diaphragm. The dome-shaped muscle located at the bottom of the lungs, used in breathing.

Diastolic blood pressure. The lower number in a blood pressure reading that represents the pressure inside the arteries when the heart is filling up with blood between contractions.

Diuretic. A medication that increases the rate that urine is produced, promoting the excretion of salts and water.

Doppler ultrasound. A test that uses high-frequency sound waves to measure blood flow through the arteries and veins.

Echocardiography. A diagnostic technique using ultrasound waves to image the interior of the heart.

Eclampsia. Onset of seizures in a pregnant woman with pre- eclampsia.

Electrocardiogram (EKG or ECG). A cardiovascular test that records the electrical impulses produced by the heart.

Heart attack. A condition that occurs when an area of the heart muscle does not receive adequate blood supply and is caused, most commonly, by coronary artery blockages.

Heart failure. Failure of the heart to pump blood with normal efficiency, causing inadequate blood flow to other organs such as the brain, liver, and kidneys. This condition can be related to a cardiomyopathy and has previously been called congestive heart failure.

High-density lipoprotein (HDL). So-called good cholesterol containing mostly protein and less cholesterol and triglycerides; high levels are associated with lower risk of coronary heart disease.

Hypertension. A chronic condition of abnormally high blood pressure.

Insulin resistance. A condition where the body is unable to properly respond to the insulin it makes. This can cause blood sugar to become elevated. Sometimes called prediabetes.

Ischemia. Decreased blood flow to the heart, brain, or other critical organs usually caused by narrowing or obstruction of an artery.

Lipids. Fatty substances (including cholesterol and triglycerides) that are found in blood and tissues.

Lipid profile. A series of blood tests used as a screening tool for abnormalities in cholesterol and triglycerides.

Lipoprotein. A particle found in blood that is a combination of lipid (fat) and protein.

Low-density lipoprotein (LDL). So-called bad cholesterol. High levels are associated with increased risk of coronary heart disease.

Menopause. Twelve months after menstruation ceases. The average age of menopause in the United States is fifty-one years.

Metabolic syndrome. Several conditions that, when they occur together, increase risk of heart disease, stroke, and diabetes. These conditions include high blood pressure, high blood sugar, excess body fat surrounding the waist (apple shape), and abnormal triglyceride levels.

Monounsaturated fats. Considered the healthy fats. Liquid at room temperature and solid when chilled, these include such fats as olive, avocado, and other nut oils.

Myocardial infarction. A blockage of blood flow to the heart muscle, causing damage to heart muscle cells. Also called heart attack.

Myocardial ischemia. Lack of oxygen-carrying blood in an area of heart tissue usually due to blocked coronary arteries. Myocardial ischemia can cause chest pain, but it also can be painless. Without intervention, myocardial ischemia can lead to a heart attack.

Myocardium. The middle and thickest layer of heart muscle.

Nuclear stress test. Uses a radioactive tracer and a special camera to evaluate the blood flow to the heart during exercise and at rest. A nuclear scan can indicate whether there is active ischemia or evidence of a scar, which usually results from a previous heart attack.

Oxygen-free radicals. Toxic chemicals released during the process of cellular respiration and released in excessive amounts as a cell dies.

Pacemaker. An electrical device that controls the heartbeat and heart rhythm by emitting a series of electrical charges.

Palpitations. The feeling that the heart is fluttering, beating too fast or irregularly, or skipping a beat.

Pericarditis. An inflammation or swelling of the membrane surrounding the heart.

Pericardium. The membrane surrounding the heart.

Polyunsaturated fats. Fat molecules that have more than one unsaturated carbon bond. Oils that contain polyunsaturated fats are typically liquid at room temperature but become solid when chilled. Polyunsaturated fats can help reduce blood cholesterol levels.

Peripheral artery disease. A condition where the arteries to the legs, arms, and other organs have narrowed. It can lead to pain and loss of function.

Plaque. Fatty substances including cholesterol, cellular waste products, calcium, and fibrin (a clotting material in the blood) that build up in the lining of an artery.

Platelet. A colorless disk-shaped body in blood that aids clotting.

Prediabetes. A condition where blood sugar is high but not so high as to be classified as type 2 diabetes. Sometimes referred to as impaired glucose tolerance.

Preeclampsia. A complication of pregnancy characterized by high blood pressure and signs of damage to another organ system, often the kidneys.

Prehypertension. A newly defined condition of having blood pressure between 120/80 and 139/89 mm Hg. This represents a warning sign that one is at higher risk of developing high blood pressure in the future.

Premature atrial contraction (PAC). Extra, abnormal heartbeats originating in the atrium that disrupt regular heart rhythm. PACs can feel like a flip-flop or skipped beat in the chest.

Premature ventricular contraction (PVC). Extra, abnormal heartbeats originating in the ventricle that disrupt regular heart rhythm. PVCs can feel like a flip-flop or skipped beat in the chest.

Protein. Amino acid compound that the body uses for growth and repair. Foods that supply the body with protein include animal products, grains, legumes, and vegetables.

Pulmonary artery. Artery carrying deoxygenated blood from the heart to the lungs.

Pulse. Measure of the heart rate. A rhythmical throbbing of the arteries as blood is propelled through them, typically as felt in the wrists or neck.

Pulse foods. A pulse is an edible seed that grows in a pod. Pulses include all beans, peas and lentils. They are low-fat sources of protein, fiber, vitamins, and minerals, and they count toward the recommended five daily portions of fruit and vegetables.

Saturated fat. Fat found in dairy products and meat; it contributes to raised cholesterol levels.

Silent ischemia. Ischemia without any pain or symptoms.

Spontaneous coronary artery dissection (SCAD). A rare condition where a sudden tear forms in the wall of a coronary artery. This results in ischemia and can cause a heart attack, abnormal heart rhythm, or death.

Statin. Any one of a class of drugs that reduce levels of LDL.

Stenosis. An abnormal narrowing of a blood vessel.

Stent. A tiny, expandable coil that is placed inside a blood vessel at the site of a blockage and then expanded to open up the blockage.

Stroke. Loss of muscle function, vision, sensation, or speech caused by either a hemorrhage or an insufficient supply of blood to part of the brain. This may be due to narrowing of the arteries supplying blood to the brain. A hemorrhage may involve bleeding into the brain itself or the space around the brain.

Systolic blood pressure. The top number in a blood pressure reading, which is a measure of the pressure inside the arteries as the heart contracts.

Tachycardia. A rapid heartbeat. Sometimes this is a normal response to exercise, anxiety, or fever. In some cases, the rapid heart rate is an abnormal response.

Takotsubo cardiomyopathy. Also known as "broken heart syndrome," this is a temporary condition that occurs as a result of acute weakening of the left ventricle, and is usually related to severe emotional or physical stress.

Total serum cholesterol. A combined measurement of a person's high-density lipoprotein (HDL), low-density lipoprotein (LDL), and triglycerides.

Triglycerides. Fats carried through the bloodstream to tissues. Most of the body's fat is stored in the form of triglycerides for later use. Triglycerides are obtained primarily from fat in foods.

Valve. A gate or door between two chambers of the heart or between a heart chamber and a blood vessel. When a heart valve is closed, no blood should pass through.

Vascular. Pertaining to the vessels that carry blood.

Ventricles. The two lower heart chambers. These chambers are responsible for pumping blood to the lungs (right ventricle) and body (left ventricle).

Ventricular tachycardia. Electrical signals in the ventricles that are fired in a very fast and uncontrolled manner, causing the heart to quiver rather than beat and pump blood. This can deteriorate to a more rapid, irregular rhythm sometimes referred to as ventricular fibrillation.

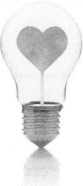

About the Authors

Jennifer H. Mieres, MD, is a Professor of Cardiology and Associate Dean of Faculty Affairs at the Zucker School of Medicine at Hofstra/ Northwell. As Senior Vice President of Northwell Health's Center for Equity of Care she has oversight of, and provides strategic guidance for, Northwell's diversity and health equity initiatives and serves as the health system's inaugural Chief Diversity and Inclusion Officer. Under Dr. Mieres's leadership Northwell Health has been recognized as a top health system for diversity, equity, and inclusion, most notably by Diversity Inc. as a "top ten" healthcare institution for a measurable commitment to healthcare justice. Northwell Health has been in the top ten list for nine consecutive years and was recognized as number one in 2020 and 2021.

A graduate of Bennington College and Boston University School of Medicine, she is a Fellow of the American Heart Association (AHA), American College of Cardiology (ACC), and Master of the American Society of Nuclear Cardiology (ASNC) and served as the first female President of the ASNC in 2009.

Dr. Mieres's clinical focus and research are centered on the elimination of health and gender disparities and cardiovascular disease in women. She is a leading advocate for patient-centered healthcare and medical education reform and has authored/coauthored over sixty-five scientific publications, including as lead author of the 2005 and 2014 AHA cardiac imaging guidelines for women. As an international speaker, she has presented her research as distinguished faculty at over a hundred forums and conferences, both nationally and internationally, including scientific sessions of the ACC, AHA, ASNC, the International Conference of Nuclear Cardiology, and IHI/BMJ International Forum on Quality & Safety in Healthcare.

A true patient and community advocate, Dr. Mieres is actively involved in service. She serves on the ACC's Diversity and Inclusion committee, is a national spokesperson for AHA's Go Red For Women movement, and has served as chair of several national AHA committees, as well as the Scientific Advisory Board for WomenHeart.

A prolific communicator, Dr. Mieres recently coauthored *Reigniting the Human Connection: A Pathway to Diversity, Inclusion, and Healthy Equity* (ForbesBooks, 2022). Her previous book, *Heart Smart for Women: Six S.T.E.P.S. in Six Weeks to Heart-Healthy Living*, was published in October 2017 along with a Spanish version, *Un Corazón Saludable para La Mujer Moderna: Seis P.A.S.O.S. en Seis Semanas para Mantener la Salud del Corazón*, in February 2019. Following her Emmy-nominated documentary, *A Woman's Heart* (2001), her creative ingenuity has evolved as an executive producer of a two-part documentary series, *Rx: The Quiet Revolution and Rx: Doctors of Tomorrow* (2015). The films have forged a change in the healthcare narrative while garnering placement on national TV network PBS and in educational institutions. She is an executive producer of the women's health documentary *Ms. Diagnosed*, which premiered at the Cinequest film festival on March 7, 2020. Dr. Mieres is routinely called upon by national and local media for expert commentary and has been designated as a most-credible voice in the healthcare industry.

A recipient of several prestigious awards, Dr. Mieres has been recognized as a tireless force fostering diversity in medical education, gender equity in cardiovascular care, as well as eliminating disparities in the delivery of healthcare to the community.

Dr. Mieres resides in New York City with her husband, Dr. Haskel Fleishaker, and their daughter, Zoë Fleishaker.

@DrJMieres
www.drjennifermieres.com

Stacey E. Rosen, MD, FACC, FACP, FAHA, is the Senior Vice President for Women's Health at the Katz Institute for Women's Health (KIWH). In this role, Dr. Rosen oversees the development and coordination of a comprehensive and integrated approach to women's health services at Northwell Health. In this role her mission has been to focus primarily on the elimination of healthcare disparities through comprehensive clinical programs, gender-based research, community partnerships, and education. She has been a practicing cardiologist for thirty years. Dr. Rosen is a Partners Council Professor of Women's Health and Professor of Cardiology at the Zucker School of Medicine at Hofstra/Northwell.

A graduate of the six-year BA-MD program at Boston University School of Medicine, Dr. Rosen is board certified in internal medicine and cardiology and is a Fellow of the American College of Cardiology, American College of Physicians, and American Heart Association.

Previously, she served as the Chief of Cardiology at Long Island Jewish Medical Center, Associate Chair of the Department of Cardiology at Northwell, and Director of the Cardiovascular Disease Fellowship at Northwell.

She has served as a longtime volunteer for the American Heart Association with leadership positions at the local, regional, and national levels and has been a national spokesperson for the AHA's Go Red for Women Movement. She served as a member of the AHA national Board of Directors, 2016–2018, and as the President, Board of Directors, Eastern States for the AHA, 2019–2021. In 2018, she received the AHA's Women in Cardiology Mentoring Award, and in 2021, she was awarded the AHA Physician of the Year, the organization's highest honor given annually to a physician who has made outstanding accomplishments in the field of cardiovascular disease.

Dr. Rosen currently serves as a member of the Scientific Advisory

Council for WomenHeart: The National Coalition for Women with Heart Disease and previously served as a member of the Roundtable on Health Literacy at the National Academy of Medicine. She coproduced her first documentary titled *Ms. Diagnosed,* which premiered at the Cinequest Film Festival on March 7, 2020.

Dr. Rosen is a recipient of numerous media, industry, and healthcare awards and is regularly called upon by the media as an expert on women's heart health.

Dr. Rosen resides in Long Island, New York, with her husband, Dr. Mark Silverman. They are the parents of three adult children, Rebecca, Max, and Sarah.

Lori M. Russo, JD, is a consultant with a focus on women's health. Prior to starting her own consulting business in 2012, Ms. Russo was in-house counsel and Americas Head of Employee Recognition and Alumni Relations for Credit Suisse, a multinational financial services company. Since 2012, Ms. Russo has concentrated on projects related to healthcare, with a specific focus on women's health and gender disparities. Recent projects include work on the two-part documentary series *Rx: The Quiet Revolution* and *Rx: Doctors of Tomorrow*, contributing author of *Heart Smart for Women: Six S.T.E.P.S. in Six Weeks to Heart-Healthy Living*, as well as coproducing the women's health documentary *Ms. Diagnosed*, which premiered at the Cinequest Film Festival on March 7, 2020. She is a graduate of Northwestern University and the Boston University School of Law.

Lori resides in New York City with her husband, Dr. Barry Shpizner. They are the parents of two adult children, Mark and Jeremy.

Marissa Licata is a registered dietitian at KIWH, where she focuses on the nutritional care of women across their life span, paying special attention to health and wellness, cardiovascular disease, gastrointestinal health, and weight management. Driven by the pursuit of helping others fulfill a healthy lifestyle and achieve nutritional wellness, Marissa has spent twenty-two years as a registered dietitian.

Prior to joining Northwell Health, Marissa had a robust career in the field of clinical nutrition, including the role of ambulatory nutrition manager at New York Presbyterian-Columbia Medical Center. She also served as Clinical Nutrition Manager of the University of California, Davis Health System, where she oversaw all aspects of clinical nutrition services among other various leading healthcare institutions. Marissa received her bachelor of science degree in food and nutrition from Long Island University, C.W. Post. She also earned her master of science degree in organizational leadership from New England College and completed her dietetic internship at New York Presbyterian-Weill Cornell Medical Center.

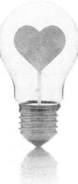

Index

F

I

J

L

M

N

Printed in the USA
CPSIA information can be obtained
at www.ICGtesting.com
JSHW011303110324
58992JS00017B/459

9 781642 252460